Hope all is well there.

Love,

Nancy

haag press

Letters from a friend with breast cancer

Compiled by Ruth Haag

Hope All Is Well There. Love, Nancy

Published by Haag Press; 315 East Market St.; Sandusky, OH 44870

Printed in the United States of America

Library of Congress Control Number : 2005927455

ISBN 0-9710260-9-2

To Nancy,

a good friend

12/21/99

Dear Ruth,

Thank you for the copies of your books you sent. I'm enjoying reading them. I'm very impressed! What alot of work. How are your sales? I also liked Bob's illustrations.

Did you ever solve the honey extractor problem? I meant to get back to you. Jason says dilute bleach is the best thing to use and then to rinse it really well. I hope I didn't already tell you this.

It has been a strange couple weeks. I found a lump in my breast just before T'giving, went to my doc who decided he couldn't feel it, but I should go for a mammogram anyway. The mammogram showed the lump & then some. I called my brother in Charlottesville & he set me up with a surgeon in C'ville who only does breasts. She (the surgeon) did a core biopsy last week and they found the lump was cancerous. So I'm scheduled for a lumpectomy - followed by radiation (to be done later in Raleigh) on Thursday. They are going to do a sentinel node procedure which should save most of my lymph nodes. After the pathology report comes back they'll decide if I need chemo. (It takes a week for it to come back.)

We are all handling it well, aside from my occasional crying jags or "sinking spells" as my sister says. We will have Christmas at my Mom's I'll have lots of family to take care of me.

Hope you have a Merry Christmas and all is well there

Love, Nancy

1/3/00

Dear Ruth,

Did Valerie & Jeremy get engaged? It's amazing how you can work things out when you try hard. Congratulations to them both!

The Catholic thing seems a bit odd but then, if she thinks that's the way to go, you can't do much about it.

I'm sure your mother will understand in time. They don't have much choice.

It was a hectic holiday. I had my lumpectomy on the 23rd. Went home to my Mom's on the 24th. On the 29th, they told me the cancer had spread farther than they thought, so I needed a mastectomy, chemo & maybe radiation. I came home to Raleigh the 31st. It had been a hard pill to swallow. My arm is still sore from the 1st surgery!

They are supposed to get back to me today for a time for the surgery. I've decided to have a bilateral mastectomy so I can have a matched set! I hope to get reconstruction at the time of surgery. We'll see if I qualify.

Jason has been a real gem. He helped me take down all the Xmas decorations & even vacuumed yesterday (I'm not supposed to do that for another week).

I do well until the sun goes down & I get tired & then I tend to fall apart. Guess that's natural.

Hope all is well there.

Love,

Nancy.

P.S. Sorry my handwriting is even worse – It's my Ⓡ arm that had surgery.

1/14/00

Dear Ruth,

Jonathan, the stuffed bear, arrived here in wonderful shape. He was glad to get out of the box. I'm glad he has experience with chemo because I don't! Thankyou!

Once again there is a twist in the road. Monday morning I had a bone scan and while I was under anesthesia Monday p.m. for my mastectomy, they got the report & saw 2 suspicious spots on my vertebrae. They woke me up without having done anything. Then I got an MRI & the next day a CAT scan. They still aren't sure what the "spots" are and they didn't feel comfortable trying to figure it out (with a bone biopsy) so I have an appointment at Duke next Thursday. We actually got in a month earlier because the drs. in Charlottesville pulled some more strings (I think they are about out of strings)

So here I sit again not knowing the plan + being zonked from the anesthesia + stress.

Otherwise things move on as usual. Hope is home sick c̄ asthma, Cole has basket ball.

Hope all is well there

Love,
Nancy +
Jonathan

1-28/00

Haags,

We are buried. North Carolina has no idea how to deal with 20 inches of snow! The roads have not been plowed or salted. There is 3 inches of ice on all the roads. We did brave it & go to a UNC vs. Univ. of MD. game last night (b'ball) It took 2 hours to get there, but it was fun.

They are playing with my tx plan again. Now it's tamoxaphen (oral) & aredia (IV - once a month) - No chemo or surgery or radiation. They found 3 spots on my vertebra. We are feeling very positive. I don't have to have chemo. We were supposed to start tx this week, but the snow shut Duke down.

I guess Jonathon wouldn't mind going for IV tx's with me!

Love, Nancy

Dear Ruth, 2/3/00

Had my first tx with Aredia on Tuesday at Duke, It was a piece of cake Good thing IV's & needles don't bother me! I am trying to be very positive. Everyone wants to know why I'm not getting chemotherapy. I just tell them it's a new thing at Duke. I keep telling myself the same thing.

I'm still thinking about what to contribute to your book of wedding advice. I think it's a great idea. When do you need it?

Hope & Cole are finally back in school today after 7 days off 2° to snow! There is still ice and snow on some of the roads.

I'm trying to make a list of all the things that didn't get done in the last six weeks that need to. I'm going to practice prioritizing big time! I think I'll cross half the things off the list!

Hope all is well there.

Love,

Nancy

To: Ruth
From: Nancy

Thanks for the wonderful foot cream. It's delightful.

Saw the following in the paper. You probably already have it but I thought it was interesting

Cole had pneumonia (very mild) & missed 3 days of school last week. He is much better.

I'm busy catching up on En Solve's books, researching vitamins, imagery & yoga classes, and getting my head on straight. The bone marrow doctor was scary. He agrees I'm not ready for that!

I'd love to help-read edit your book.

I still find it hard to be around people. I find their conversations trivial & I can't concentrate. I'm sure that will change.

Thanks for all your support.

Love, Nancy

Dear Kaags,

Happy Valentine's Day!

Thanks for all your support!

Lots of Love,

Nanay

2/29/00

Dear Ruth,

Thank you so much for the beautiful book. I've been thinking I need a book to write the inspirational & humorous things I come across.

I've been working on the cookbook. What fun! I hope to send it to you later this week along with marriage advice.

I'm at Duke right now waiting for my IV tx. You get here at nine & if you're lucky you get done by 3 or 4<u>00</u>. Jason came with me this morning so we can talk to the dr. together. He's going back to work after we see the doc. I'll stay & get my tx.

Jasons's Mom is coming Thursday. She'll be here until Monday,

I've been doing clerical work for Jason almost every morning. Nothing much gets done at home. I still don't have my energy back.

EnSolve sold it's first petroleminator to a ship. It was shipped out yesterday. It's all very exciting

Hope all is well there

Love,

Nancy

3/6/00

Dear Ruth,

The cook book is in the mail. Jason's mother left today, so I'm hoping things can get more organized.

Marriage advice.

1) If you have to fight, fight nice - Stick to the subject, Sometimes you have to put yourself in "time out" for a minute to cool off.

2) Remember you are friends and lovers above all. Go on dates, give each other little surprises, remember birthdays, anniversaries + other occasions.

3) Try to get along with your in-laws. Remember, if you are lucky you, too will be a mother or father-in-law.

4) When I asked Hope + Ole what they thought we did that enables us to stay married they both decided Compromise was the most important.

More later, Nancy

3/14/00

Dear Ruth,

I hope you got the cookbook by now. What are your other cookbooks going to be?

I am thinking about taking Hope + Cole on a "road trip" to see Steve + Debbie Ranger in Detroit. We would love to stop in Findlay on the way and see you. We don't have any dates set yet. We wondered when might be a good time for you.

I signed up for a "Mindfulness" Program at Duke yesterday. It sounds like what I need to help myself through this disease

Hope all is well there

Love, Nancy

PS. I've faxed the sheet from the program.

3/14/00

Ruth,

Hope + I loved the fire story. Neighbors can be such a pain.

I'm planning to drive to Michigan. As we call it "road trip" We will take several days to do it. Please don't worry about sleeping arrangements. We are all capable of sleeping on the floor.

I saw the following article in the paper. Here we have a status symbol + didn't know. Thought the 1st 2 paragraphs were the most interesting.

Hope you're having a good day

Love
Nancy

P.S. I finally found a nutritionist at Duke. I go to see her next week.

The great news is Jason bought a new iMac for us to use at home! It is wonder ful! It doesn't even crash when I'm on the Internet! I have a new email address:

ncaplan@ensolve.com.

Thanks for the directions. I'm looking at July 13 + 14 (arriving sometime on the 13th + leaving early on the 15th). Let me know if that works. (We're just what you need the week after the wedding - right?)

Hope all is well there.

Love

Nancy

4/5/00

Dear Ruth,

Thank you for the goodie bag of Burts' Bees. It seems like a great assortment. I'll let you know how I like every thing. There was an article in the paper about how Burts was moving out of Raleigh — I'm not sure to where though. I'd meant to cut it out.

I enjoyed your letter re: Valerie and her changing plans. I guess that's typical. Here I thought parents started Valium when they're children were in high school!

We are having guests today Kim + his second wife + her daughter Jen (she's 13). They are staying until Sunday. In my current state of mind/health getting ready for company is almost too exhausting + overwhelming! but I'm almost there.

I start my "Mindfulness" class at Duke today. That should be interesting..

Hope is about ready to go to the bus stop so I'd better go.– I walk after she leaves.

My family dr. yesterday said I should walk 2 miles instead of one. I'm not sure where to fit that in. He also looked at my shoulder +

said I had tendonitis due to
my surgery - I spend half
my life at the doc's. The other
half at the drug store.

Hope all is well there

Love,

Nancy

My new e-mail:
ncaplan@ensolve.com 4/19/00

Dear Ruth,

I can't believe Valerie is already finished for the year! We just started Spring Break. We are going to my parents tomorrow through Easter. That should be fun.

Jason + 2 of my friends had a huge surprise b'day party for me (a little early) on the 8th. I knew about it because I told Jason I wanted a party with my friends + their kids out at Beaver Dam (on Falls Lake). They had it all planned, but as soon as we arrived a huge front came through + it poured! There was a tornado about a mile away. The temperature dropped from 72° to 42° in less than 2 hours. It was fun any way. My parents came +

one of my friends flew in from Texas. (Those *were* surprises).

They gave me a day at the spa & dinner out as a gift. I was overwhelmed. I didn't want any gifts!

The only thing I've learned about photographers after watching my mom negotiate 4 weddings & a 50th anniversary party is that if you can just get them to take the pictures & give you the negatives it's much cheaper-to get made what you want. Most photographers won't do it.

I'm feeling fine other than fatigue which is probably 2° the tamoxifen. I have been walking 1¼ miles every morning since last fall. The mindfulness class is a bit of a challenge. There are some strange people in it & I've never been the "meditative-beautiful" people type. I haven't given up though.

I go back to have my tests updated April 25. Hope it's good news. Hope all is well there

Love,

Nancy

Subj: Re: Ruth trying your e-mail
Date: 4/28/00

Ruth,

I got your e-mail. My problem with e-mail is that I am a terrible typist. I guess using it was sort of like our grandparents getting used to talking on the phone long distance instead of writing. Each generation seems to have a new way to communicate.

I have been at Duke the last three days and must say I'm a bit weary. On Tuesday, I left home at 6:15 am and got home at 8:30 pm. I had a bone scan, a skeletal scan, saw the doc and had my aredia tx. The doc said the scans showed nothing different, which is actually good. He said the aredia could have made lots of other sites show up. I think one of the hardest parts of going up there is seeing all those really sick people in the waiting rooms. I have finally resigned myself to having to wait a long time for appointments, so I bring lots of things to do and make sure Hope and Cole and Jason are all taken care of for the day.

Wednesday, Jason and I went to the support group. (They have one or two sessions for men). This time was not quite as good as the last – a couple new women have joined and I'm not crazy about them.

Today, I went for Mindfulness course. I found I'm not the only one having difficulty, so that helped. I have to keep trying to convince myself this can really improve your immune system.

I also went to the paint store and picked up two other colors of paint to try on the exterior of the house. The painters are supposed to start on Monday, but is has been so wet, I think it may have to dry out for a few days. It is hard to tell what the colors will look like on the whole house. We are changing to some sort of beige/tan/gray on the house and a lighter shade of the same for the trim. We are tired of all that blue/gray trim. The shutters will be dark blue – What a surprise.

How are your house plans coming? Haven't heard for a while.

More on photographers. I know a couple people who had friends that were interested in photography take pictures at their weddings. It freed up the family to enjoy the wedding.

Guess I better run, I have to get a few errands done. For some reason this family likes to have food in the house and clean laundry.

Hope all is well there.

Love,

Nancy

Subj: <no subject>
Date: 5/19/00
May 18, 2000

Dear Ruth,

It has been a sad two weeks. The 9 year old boy, from our neighborhood, who has been sick with complications from strep since January, died. One of the boys who used to mow our lawn (they moved to Texas a couple years ago), died in a car accident. He would have been 18 in a week. A nine year old boy whose grandfather works at Cole's school disappeared in January. His mother's boyfriend was suspected of taking him, but the guy wouldn't talk. Anyway, they found the boy in a suitcase, last week. One of the guys that goes fishing with Jason in the fall died this week. We are all holding our breath.

Cole is having nightmares every night. Can't imagine why. He wants to know why everyone that has died is male.

The school year is winding down I guess. I'm not quite ready for it to be out. I've been working for Jason more. I'm the "Girl Friday". It seems to take some of the burden off of him. My mother says, "Who is doing your job" and I told her no one. I will have to get more organized if I plan to keep this up.

Hope all is going well with the wedding plans. Are they going on a honeymoon?

Better get going on the company books.

Hope all is well there.
Love,
Nancy

Subj: Onward
Date: 5/23/00

Dear Ruth,

Things are a bit better, though I had a bout with a bad UTI and it took me 12 hours to get the docs to call in a script! And 4 days to feel better. I keep saying I should have gone to medical school just so I could write my own scripts. I'm finally feeling better.

I got the nicest package in the mail. Thank you for the drawer liners. I don't wear cologne or use much soap, because I've become allergic to most of it, but I always keep my drawers lined with paper. At least my undies smell nice. I needed some new paper. My old stuff was mille fleur by Crabtree and I don't think they even make it any more.

I went for another Aredia tx today. I didn't have to see the doc, so I was home by 11:00.

Cole and Hope's soccer tournament was last weekend – Cole's team came in 2nd (They should have been 1st, but the coach messed up big time). We won't comment on Hope's team. Let's just say they have fun. We had 8 games altogether. I only went Sunday.

Someone called me this morning and asked me how I was doing and I said fine and she said that's what she thought, but that she had been told by Cole's coach that I was terminal, they had tried everything and had given up on me! Nice thing to hear. I have a call in to someone to straighten him out. It's hard enough to be positive without that.

The painters came today to power wash the house. It looks

better already. They are to start painting on Friday. It's very exciting.

I am going to Chicago (did I tell you this?) on June 4 to see a doc who is supposed to specialize in complementary medicine, esp. nutrition and supplements. It's a long story how I got to him, anyway, It's the Block Medical Center in Evanston, IL. They are on the web.

The pool is open and Cole wants to go every day. They have end of grade tests this week, so there is no homework. Hope has a field trip to the beach to see salt marches, etc. on Friday. Of course, I volunteered for that one. I'm riding with another parent, not on the bus.

Hope all is well there.

Love,

Nancy

Subj: Every Day a Letter from Ruth?
Date: Tues, May 23, 2000

Nancy,

Bob and I are traveling to Chicago on June 1 for a book publisher's conference. We will be starting for home on June 4. Your news of being in Chicago on the same day is exciting! Do you want us to meet with you somewhere? Do you need a ride from the airport? Do you need support with your doctor's visit? Isn't the world small? Let us know if we can be any sort of assistance. Bob will be back in the Chicago area on June 7.

Much love,

Ruth

Re: Every Day a Letter From Ruth?
Date: 5/28/00
Dear Ruth,

I just got back from the cub scout campout. I survived though I need a long nap. I'm too old to sleep on the ground.

What a small world is right. I think my plane comes in around 9 or 10 am. I don't know when you plan to leave. Could we meet for brunch/lunch? I'm supposed to be staying at the Holiday Inn in Evanston. There are supposed to be some nice places to eat in Evanston. I planned to take a shuttle from the airport.

Love,

Nancy

Subj: Are you sure?

Date: 5/31/00

Dear Ruth,

I would love to see you, but are you sure you want to go so far out of your way? My flight arrives at O'Hare Airport at 9:20 am. It's American Airline flight #1703.

How long does it take for you to get home from Chicago? Is Rachel or Val going with you?

Both Hope and Cole are home sick today. Cole has a sore throat and Hope has her usual cold with asthma. The painters were here, a man was here to cut down a couple of trees and I had three appointments today and I was supposed to help at Jason's office. Too much for one day. I cancelled all but my haircut (we must prioritize) and left Hope in charge while I went to help at the office.

All is calmer now.

Much love,

Nancy

Subj: Re: Are you sure?
Date: 5/31/00

Nancy,

We'll be there Sunday morning at O'Hare. It takes us about 6 hours to get home, so we will deliver you, get you settled, eat something and then start for home.

Much love,

Ruth

Subj: Can't wait!
Date: 5/31/00

Dear Ruth,

That will be great! My mom is very concerned about me traveling by myself. I'm not a very seasoned solo traveler. She kept trying to convince me to have her come with me. (I guess moms never stop worrying.) She was very pleased to hear you might meet me.

See you Sunday! What a nice extra to get to see you!

Much love,

Nancy

Subj: Thanks!
Date: 6/9/00

Dear Ruth and Bob,

It was so good to see you last Sunday. Thanks again for rescuing me from the airport. My visit went well. They were very positive and advised me to follow a diet that consists of everything I don't like to eat and nothing I do – or so it seemed. It's a basic no meat, no dairy, no sugar, no refined flour diet. They also prescribed a bunch of vitamins and supplements. I ordered them, but the cost is prohibitive and so we will have to work that out. The docs and dietician were very helpful and supportive. Wish we had them in Raleigh. Actually they said they were considering opening a clinic here in Chapel Hill, but they hadn't found a doc yet to run it. I took the "el" to the airport and got home safe and sound about 10:30 Monday night.

I have been trying to get ready to go to the beach on Sunday, but there have been lots of distractions and obstacles – mostly the painters – they finished today and we are very pleased. It looks like a new house. I had to make another trip to the paint store yesterday after they put up the color I had picked and found out it was awful! I finally found the blue I wanted. It's called "Old Navy", which I find amusing since that is Hope's favorite store.

Cole's school called me yesterday and said he had hurt his wrist. I got him and after the crazed trip to the paint store, took him to the doc and they said to x-ray it. So we did. Thank goodness it is just sprained. He has a splint they gave him. It was hard not to have the materials to make one for him myself, but I guess I'm a bit out of practice.

Hope's graduation was this morning. It was very nice – an

hour and then they came home at 9:30 am. Those girls are scary the way they look. They all look about 18.

I have been trying to finish the company books for May tonight, but I'm too tired and so I'm going to call it a night.

Hope all is well there.

Much love,

Nancy

Subj: How was it?
Date: 7/8/00

Dear Ruth,

How was the wedding????? We thought about you all day on the fourth. Can't wait to hear all about it. Did Valerie and Jeremy go on a honeymoon? Hope all went well.

Also, were you recovered enough to celebrate your anniversary? Twenty five years is quite a milestone.

My nephews, Russ and Rob (They are Cole's age), have been here all week. It has been fun having triples, but I'm tired. We went to the Mudcats (baseball) for the Fourth, to the new science museum Thursday, out tubing on the boat Thursday night and to the Four Tops and Beach Boys concert last night. They are supposed to go home today. Their dad is flying his plane to pick them up.

Tonight I'm driving to VA to pick up Hope. She is with my other sister at Mountain Lake – a resort in the mountains. We decided it was too far for me to drive in one day, so I'm going to stay in a motel tonight. I think I could use the rest.

We are all very excited about our trip next week. We still plan to be at your place on Thursday late afternoon. I'll call with a more specific time when I figure it out.

Hope all is peaceful and well.

Love,

Nancy

Subj: A Quickie
Date: 7/9/00

Ruth,

Thanks for the note. I just got back from picking up Hope and I'm trying to finish the books for Jason today.

Re: Hope's likes and dislikes. They are both what I call selective eaters. I tell people please do not worry about what they will eat. I always tell Hope and Cole they can have cereal for dinner if they don't like what we're having and I always travel with their favorites. Also please don't make yourself crazy figuring out what I can eat. I'm getting adaptable, but yes I can have olive and canola oil.

More later.

Love,

Nancy

Subj: Thanks
Date: 7/11/00

Dear Ruth,

Thank you for the road closing warning. I guess even Ohio has, as Jason's sister says, "Exit du jour" – of course she lives in Washington.

I also got this wonderful book in the mail yesterday. What a beautiful book! We were all very impressed. I keep meaning to tell you I met a woman at the airport in Chicago. She has worked for Algonquin Books in Chapel Hill for 7 years and is now starting her own business. She plans to market individual books. I doubt you are interested but I told her I would give you her name.

We are all so excited about our trip. I think we'll get to your place somewhere between 4 and 5pm on Thursday. I'll let you know if that changes.

Oh, I told Cole you had a pond to swim in. He thought for a minute and said "I wonder if there are fish in that pond." I told him I would ask. He is his father's son.

Love,

Nancy

Subj: Thanks
Date: 7/21/00

Dear Bob and Ruth,

Thanks for looking after my family. They had a great time! Cole was absolutely ecstatic about his fishing success in your pond. Hope enjoyed seeing the hospital she was born in and our old house on 1st Street.

Thanks again!

Regards,

Jason

7/26/00

Dear Ruth,

We are finally back home for a couple days! We go to VA. on Friday for the weekend.

We all so enjoyed our visit with you. Thanks for every thing - Touring us around town, the Wonderful lunch, the morning walks, the great company + especially for finding food I could eat! Can't forget the fishing!

We enjoyed Michigan and went to Canada for one day.

Last weekend we went to Lake Gaston with some friends (There were

20 of us) We had a great time between 3 boats c̄ tubes + 2 jet ski even though the weather was gloomy.

I only rode in the boat. I gave up tubing + jet skis ~ too scary. Cole caught a huge catfish. He was pleased.

I am trying to clean out my pantry today + go to the health food store.

Hope all is well there.

Love,

Nancy

Subj: <no subject>
Date: 8/10/00
Dear Ruth,

I think the kids are more ready than I am for school. School starts on Monday. I don't like getting up before 6 am. Hope's school starts at 7:30 and Cole's doesn't start until 9:15. That's a pain.

Cole is not very enthusiastic re: school because the reputation the teachers he has is they give a ton of homework, hard tests and are not very flexible. Unfortunately the rumors are mostly true. His two teachers have been there for at least ten years (which is when Hope started there) and the scoop has been the same. He should learn a lot, if they don't make him crazy first.

Hope is looking forward to school, if only because she will get to see her friends. They are coming back together after many of them were split up in elementary and middle school.

They are both sick this week. Cole has a cold. Hope has a full blown asthma episode. I saw a nurse practitioner who didn't know us. After we started to tell her about Hope's history, she said, "Oh I know you, you're Hope, I know about you." They gave her a "breathing tx" and were a bit concerned. They changed some of her meds and gave her new ones. I think she's finally turning the corner. I can't even consider letting her out of the house when the weather is like this. Hopefully she'll be better by Monday.

Jason and I are busy planning our trip to Europe. We leave the 14th and are going to Switzerland, Germany and France. We are going to ride the train everywhere. It will be an adventure, since neither of us has ever been to Europe before. We will be gone two weeks. We are having fun trying to communicate re: reservations over the Internet, via fax and telephone. I get a kick out of Jason talking to them over the phone. Of course I'm not brave enough to try it myself. I went to the mall this morning to get a few things for Jason for his B'day. I found 2 silk polo shirts and micro-fiber slacks on sale that should work great for the trip. Also found a few other little gadgets like a new Swiss army knife (he lost his) and a compass on a key ring. We plan to carry just one bag each that each weighs 20 lbs. We'll have to pack light.

Got our photos back from the trip. I plan to go through them in the next week or two and send a few to you. The fish were impressive.

Hope all is well there. When does school start?

Love,

Nancy

Subj: Rough Start
Date: 8/21/00

Dear Ruth,

Last week was a bust, especially since it was the first week of school! First, my Aunt Dora died on Friday night. She was the one with nine kids and the daughter named Ruth. I liked her a lot. I spent the weekend trying to figure out a way to get to her funeral which was on Tuesday. I didn't make it.

Cole woke up in the middle of the night, Sunday, with terrible ear pain. He didn't even make it to school on the first day. I took him to the doctor and they said he had swimmer's ear.

Hope's bus came at 6:05, 6:25, 7:00, 6:30 and not at all one day. This is going to be tough. Hope's school starts at 7:30 and she gets home at 2:45. Cole's school doesn't start until 8:45 and he gets home at 4:15. I can't figure out when he can get in homework and playtime with his friends (which I think is important). I guess I'll get used to it.

I found out one of our neighbors has pancreatic cancer.

My nephew Noah had surgery on Monday. He went home on Thursday, only to go back on Saturday. My sister is exhausted and a bit beside herself.

Tuesday I spent the day at Duke. I don't mind the treatment. I just have a hard time with seeing all the sick people. Wednesday, I went to the support group at Duke. It's good, but only a few came.

Friday Cole got sick again, so I picked him up at school. He said he hasn't felt well all week. This morning he said he hated school and wasn't going back. It was too boring. He went. I'll have to pay more attention to see what's going on. I think he is just scared of the work that they supposedly get in fourth grade.

By the end of the week everyone was mad and out of sorts.

The weekend was much better. We cut down a lot of branches that were blocking our view of the street and trimmed the bushes. Jason figured out what clothes he is going to take to Europe. Hope and I went to Border's.

Today I spent the morning remaking and hemming some clothes I got on a great sale, but of course I felt they needed more work. (added a pocket, made the legs narrower, let out the waistband, etc.) I finished all 7 things.

We have our plans all made for the trip. I am getting quite excited. I almost have my suitcase packed and we don't leave until the 14th.

I'm sure this week will go better. I have a book club tonight. We are discussing The Poisonwood Bible.

Hope all is well there,

Love,

Nancy

Subj: Busy
Date: 9/11/00

Dear Ruth,

Even though I thought I was being very organized about getting ready for the trip, I still have a bunch of things to do. Part of the problem was Cole being sick last week. He has not really felt well since school started. Last week I took him in to the doctor for the third time since school started once for swimmer's ear, once for stomach pain and once for fever and coughing and they finally gave him some antibiotics. The doc wanted to know if Cole was an asthmatic because he was wheezing and I said he wasn't allowed to be one. He is finally feeling better. Now we have a ton of make-up work to do.

I got all my stuff into my backpack and it weighs 17 pounds. (I have a self imposed limit of 20), so I can add my last minute things.

Hope is really liking high school. I thought she would. She has lots of friends and likes actually learning, instead of having the teachers having to spend half their time on discipline. I went to her Open House last week and met all her teachers. They all seem great, except her Civics teacher, who is very boring.

I guess I'd better get cleaning.

Love,

Nancy

9/16/00

Dear Ruth,

We are actually in Switzer-
land & it feels so unbelieve-
able. It really looks
like the photo! The mountain
views, the f lowers & the
food are fantastic! Our
room has a balcony &
overlooks the Alps. They
are impressive. We even
had a sauna today. Hiked
a trail & didn't see another
tourist. Hope all is
well there, Lots of Love, Nancy

Subj: It was great!
Date: 10/10/00

Dear Ruth,

Yes, we are back. We had a great time. The food was wonderful. The scenery was beautiful. The people were friendly. The company was the best. We loved the trains. I'll have to send you a photo or two when they come in.

It was back to reality in a big way though. I went to Duke on Thursday and they did another bone scan. The doc said it looked like there might be signs of healing in the tumor in my L-1 vertebrae, but he wants to do another x-ray next month – sigh.

Hope is enjoying high school. Report cards come out next week. Cole says he hates school and wants to be home schooled. I have a meeting with the gifted teacher this week. I think he is just bored. I talked to the principal last week and asked her if there should be an advanced math group in Cole's class and she said, "Isn't there?" Cole came home Friday and told that they had just formed a new math group – squeaky wheels.

The kids had a soccer tournament over the weekend. I hate them, but Hope and Cole love them. Hope played 4 games and Cole 3. Both of their teams lost.

I'm trying to get the books done for September, but I'm not very motivated. It is much more fun surfing the net. I've been Christmas shopping that way.

I have to get moving. I wasn't supposed to work in the library at Cole's school today, but they called and asked if I could sub, so I said yes – silly me.

More later.

Hope all is well there. Congratulations on your book sale!

Love,

Nancy

Subj: No time
Date: 10/25/00

Dear Ruth,

I'm still trying to find the two hours that I lost with Hope and Cole's new school schedules. Hope leaves at 6:30, Cole at 9:00 and Hope gets home at 2:40 and Cole at 4:15. I think Hope needs an after school activity at school. It seems their activities are taking up more time, too. Cole is only doing soccer and cub scouts and Hope is doing soccer and did I tell you? – girl scouts! There is a troop of 5 girls from the neighborhood in the troop. They call it "that thing." They don't want their friends to know about it. The leader is a friend of mine and a wonderful person. They have a lot of fun things planned. I have been trying to find something for Hope to get interested in other than soccer.

They got report cards today. Hope hasn't missed a day of school. They both got one B and the rest A's. Cole told me one of his friend's sister was getting a scooter because she got all A's. I explained we don't believe in that – that grades are their own reward and he said he knew that. He just wanted to know why other parents would do that.

We went to an ice hockey game last night with one of the organizations Jason belongs to. It was lots of fun. Most of the people stood around talking (they had a suite). I was quite happy, because I got to watch the game in great seats and no one bugged me.

I went to Charlottesville last weekend to see my sister Julie. She was trying to find curtains for her guest room. She does not decorate, but has a gorgeous garden. We were successful and found some she likes and hung them. I also found a frame I was looking for and finished the handwork on Hope and Cole's lap quilts I'm making them for Xmas. Jason, Hope and Cole went camping Sat. night with some neighbors and had a great time.

Guess I better run. Jason' mom is coming Friday.

Hope all is well there.

Love,

Nancy

Subj: I'm not lost
Date: 11/9/00

Dear Ruth,

I told everyone I was answering e-mail and to leave me alone for a little while. I doubt it will work. Cole has missed 3 days of school (Weds, Fri and Mon. They were off on Tues.). He had a sinus infection, started on antibiotics and then went to school Friday. I thought he had eaten breakfast. He hadn't and threw up all over his classroom on Friday. There is a bad stomach bug going around and so on Monday when he was going to throw up I wasn't about to send him! I called the doc and they want to finish the antibiotics. (I thought we should try a different one. What do mothers know?)

I went to Duke on Thursday. The doc said the x-ray was about what he thought. The tumor is not smaller, but there is some bone being laid down inside it. He also decided to change my medication from Tamoxifen to Arimidex. I was thrown for quite a loop. He said he didn't like that the tumor markers were still going up, which is what Jason and I have been saying for the last few months. I had read that when one hormone stops working they try another and a few more and if that doesn't work they do chemo. I got a little ahead of myself. The best is that Arimidex was just approved for patients like me and my brother says that the doc was just "upgrading my computer."

I also took Hope to the dermatologist on Tuesday (for her second visit.) The doc removed a bunch of plugs from Hope's pores. She said, "I told you about this last time, right?" We said, "No." Anyway the bottom line is that it will take six months of treatment and after that topical meds should take care of it. I wish I'd know before, I would have taken her a year ago!

Not having a great week with docs!

I did put aside everything and make Jason a shirt for Christmas the last couple of days. My sister made him one when we were first married. He has been asking for one like it for the last couple of years. I decided to call my sister and see if she still had the pattern and she did! It is a flannel shirt with a neckband and a four button placket down the front and no cuffs – just roll up sleeves. He'll be surprised. Hope it's like he remembers. It looks a bit dated to me.

They called yesterday and Hope is going to start Driver's Ed on Monday. I think I am the only one who is excited…Hope and I talked about it and we decided she is just very scared. I told her I'd take her up to the school and let her drive Jason's truck for a little bit. She thought that was a great idea. I think she doesn't want to be embarrassed. Driver's Ed is three hours a day for 2 weeks after school. You have to have your learner's permit for a year before you can get your license and you have to be 15 and have Driver's Ed to get your learner's. I'm sure it will be a year before Jason lets her out of the driveway.

Guess I'm being called for Math help. More later (Hopefully sooner than last time).

Hope all is well there.

Love,

Nancy

Subj: Turkey Week
Date: 11/21/00

Dear Ruth,

Thank you for the little snowman. We all agree he's (she's) very cute. Can you believe we got 2 inches of snow yesterday? It's the earliest snow here for 30 years. We had a great time in the hot tub (we always go in in the snow). School was on a 2 hour delay today. The snow is nearly gone now.

Hope started Driver's Ed (the written part), I have taken her up to Cole's school to let her try driving my car. She did very well. I think it will take a lot of practice before I feel comfortable. Apparently, they don't go on a track like we did. They start right out on the road!!!!! How scary. I'm going to watch Driver's Ed cars more carefully now.

Cole would love to join Rachel being home schooled. He really dislikes his teachers and is alternately bored and scared he'll do something wrong. I went in and talked to them Friday. Maybe it will do some good. They didn't have any idea he was unhappy. I finally told Cole I couldn't home school him because I didn't know enough. We would both be miserable. Sounds like a great idea for Rachel though if she's bored. How is Val doing in school?

I'm getting ready to go to my Mom's. Of course Jason is going to the Outer Banks with his crew. It actually works out well. He gets very bored at my parents. Somehow I agreed to let Hope bring a friend with her to Charlottesville. The one I thought was coming couldn't and so Hope found an alternate. I like her. Should be nice for Hope to have a girl to hang out with for a change. Usually there are only boy cousins around most of the time. My mother is quite pleased. She loves a house full. Sometimes I wonder if I'm related.

We are going to the high school B'ball game tonight – at least Cole and I are. Hope and Jason aren't sure, yet. Party Poopers.

My new medicine seems to make me even more tired. I will have more blood work done on December 7. It is a bit scary when I get really tired because I'm always afraid it's the disease and not the medicine. One day at a time.

Hope all is well there.

Happy Thanksgiving.

Love,

Nancy

Subj: No, it wasn't
Date: 12/4/00

Ruth,

I mail my Xmas cards every year the day after Thanksgiving from my mother's house. I just hate that job, so I do it first. I couldn't decide what to write, so I just sent the letter and didn't write any little notes like I usually do. I have about finished doing my shopping. I was going to bake this week, but Hope now has a full blown asthma episode and is home. We watched "Holiday Affair" this morning (with Robert Mitchum and Janet Leigh). That was after I went to the office and paid bills for Jason.

We were supposed to get 20 inches of snow on Sunday!! We barely got ½". Everyone here was going crazy on Saturday. I went out at 8 am to find some boots for Cole. He had outgrown the ones from last year and we were debating on whether he really needed them this year. Many years we don't get any snow. Needless to say Cole was very upset that they had school today. He tries to find any excuse not to go.

I went to Duke three times last week. Once for a mammogram. I don't want to even discuss it except they gave me a hard time and kept asking about what they saw along the scar line. I went to my support group Wednesday night and heard a woman speak who has been battling cancer (I hate that phrase, but haven't found a better one yet) for 12 years. She was quite remarkable. I went Thursday for my treatment and to see my doc. I asked him about seeing a plastic surgeon about having the lumps and bumps taken out of my scar and he said he thought it was a great idea. I see the plastics guy tomorrow. He did his fellowship at Sloan Kettering (They are the #1 cancer center in the country). He should know what he's doing. I'm only going to TALK to him. Last December was enough of a nightmare. We don't need any more of that this year.

We got the tree up. It is the same one we bought in Findlay after our house almost caught on fire. It's looking a bit shabby. I think we may have to get a new one next year.

I love the robe you sent me last year. Every time I put it on Cole says "That is so soft. Who sent it to you – Your cousin Ruth or the Ruth with the pond?" I say, "Ruth Haag, the one with the pond." And he proceeds to talk all about how much fun he had catching fish there last summer.

Guess I'd better get to work on November books. Speaking of books – Do you know about Half.com? they have used books for a song. I taught my dad how to Internet shop on that site over Thanksgiving. Hope all is well there.

Love,

Nancy

P.S . Would your parents enjoy the exhibit at Findlay College that we saw?

Subj: <no subject>
Date: 12/7/00

Dear Ruth,

Tuesday was what I call a stupid day. I went to see the plastics guy. He said that it's not scar tissue and he didn't know what it was and I need to see one of the breast surgeons. That I wasted a whole day on – while Hope was home sick. I think my time would have been better spent making Christmas cookies and watching movies with Hope. They have me scheduled to see the surgeon on the 20th. I really think they want to biopsy the thing and see what it is. The scar line itself is well healed. It's just the lumps that bug me. Tell Bob thanks for the advice on the medicine, however it seemed that I will always be on some kind of Rx. I got the last value for the tumor marker and it's still going up –not what we wanted. The doc said it would take another 3 or 4 weeks before they know if this new med is working.

The 14th is the anniversary of my first diagnosis, so I'm as my sister Susan says a bit "wiggy." I hope to start baking today. I think instead of the usual blitz, I'm going to try a batch a day.

Jason is in New Orleans until Friday. I seem to have been chosen to take care of work problems. I try to stay out of it, but sometimes it doesn't work.

Cole is wanting to know about all kinds of things that have escaped me – like Pi, bell curves, the IQ's of people like Einstein and others. In the meantime he needs to learn how to add fractions! I guess I'll have to get to the library or get on the net to get some simplified info for him. Got any good resources for a nine year old who is a bit ahead of his time? His librarian at school is trying, but she's of little help. The

AG teacher is rarely there. So I guess it's up to Cole and me. He found an old Consumer Report book the other day and I think he thought he was in heaven.

Hope is recovering well from her latest bout of asthma.

Hope all is well there.

Love,

Nancy

Subj: Wow!
Date: 12/14/00

Dear Ruth,

Thanks so much for the gorgeous roses. They are especially pretty because they put winter greens in with the usual ferns. It was just what I needed. I'm driving myself crazy lately worrying. My back has been hurting, but I think we have decided it is muscular from all of the Xmas stuff I do that I'm not used to. I went in the hot tub this morning and that helped.

I have almost finished baking cookies and have some wrapping left to do. Hope has exams next week and will only have half days. We are trying to figure out if the busses will run.

Cole is busy working on another stupid book report. I don't know why they can't just write the thing and not have to decorate a paper bag vest with illustrations from the book, and buttons and sequins.

I am going to an ornament party tonight and a neighborhood party on Saturday. They should be fun and put me in the Christmas spirit. I do dread getting cornered by well meaning people that say in this weird voice, "How are you doing?" I can't decide if they want to hear "Just fine" or the gory details. I usually go with, " just fine".

Sorry to hear about your nephew. I wonder if your sister listens to Dr. Laura. That's what she would have advised. Some parents around here think that calling the police is a good idea. I'm not so sure. I think I would go the counseling route. I hope your roof is holding. They keep telling us we are going to get sleet and we get a few sprinkles of rain.

Guess I better get Cole off to school. Hope all is well (and dry) there. Thanks again for the flowers.

Love,

Nancy

Title: Bells
Yahoo Greetings

Merry Christmas!

We are off to Washington and Virginia on Tuesday.
More when we return.
Hope you have a wonderful holiday.
Lots of love.

-Nancy

Subj: Re: Hello? Are you there?
Date 1/17/01

Ruth,

This is Jason. I promise I won't read your e-mail to Nancy but I wanted to let you know that we are having a bit of trouble reading e-mail at home so Nancy has not been able to respond. Her operation went well yesterday. They cut out a bit more of her breast tissue than they thought they were going to but they said it went well. She starts chemotherapy next week (Monday) for the first of three installments. I have to run now but will fill you in on the details later. Thanks for your support.

Jason

Subj: Cozy
Date: 1/30/01

Ruth,

Thanks for the cozy socks. They are wonderful. As you can see, Jason got the e-mail working again. I'm almost able to read a page or two. Typing is a real challenge. I'm doing better. My chest has been quite sore where they put in the Hickman, but it's healing.

My new cleaning lady comes tomorrow. Jason keeps trying to figure out why I'm trying to straighten up for her. I keep explaining there is a difference between cleaning and straightening so you can clean. Cole is also puzzled. Hope understands. Guess it's a guy thing.

More later when my head clears more. I have a bad case of "chemo brain."

Love,

Nancy

Subj: FW: Nancy's necklace
Date: 2/6/01

Ruth,

Thank you for the soup mix. It looks delicious. My kind of cooking! I am feeling much better. My sisters were here for the weekend. They got me all fixed up with hats, scarves and my wig. I had my head shaved last Wednesday. It's amazing how easy it is to be bald. I can get ready very quickly in the morning. There is no water dripping down my neck after a shower and I save so much money on shampoo and electricity since I don't have to dry and curl my hair – right. I got brave and wore my skull cap and scarf all day even shopping. I hardly got any stares.

Hope is taking the driving part of Driver's Ed. She doesn't really like it. She says her teacher is mean. She has it one more night – 5:45 to 8:45. Then she can get her permit.

They are starting a new support group at Duke tomorrow for breast cancer patients with "Chronic Disease" – much better than metastatic disease. It is a breakfast meeting. Since I've been requesting this group I guess I'd better go.

The forwarded photo is one of the necklace my family gave me. They each picked out or made a charm for it. Hope you can retrieve it.

Hope all is well there.

Love,

Nancy

Subj: House of Cards
Date: 2/11/01

Dear Ruth,

We are in danger of the "House of Cards" tumbling. I'm to get my treatment tomorrow. There is an ice storm predicted tonight (the kids are off school, at least). Hope has a cold/ sore throat and a tight chest. Cole sprained his ankle Wednesday (It's now getting better). The rescue team is coming today (my mom and dad). I told Jason I'm feeling selfish. I want to feel sick by myself and not take care of everyone else.

The good news is Hope passed her Driver's Ed and can now get her permit once she gets a note from school that says she is passing. In NC, if you are failing school they take away your license. Hopefully, Jason will take her this week to get it. She has to pass a written test to get it.

Jason and Cole had their last regular season B'ball game last night. Their record is 5 and 3, which is quite amazing considering how young the team is. I didn't go because Cole wasn't playing and I don't want to be around all those germy people. Now soccer starts for both of them. At least their practice field is only 10 minutes away and easy to get to. The good thing about soccer is that it is outside, so I can stay away from all the germs. I think I'm beginning to sound paranoid.

I'd love to read your new book. I'm thinking about writing a book about ways to cover bald heads when this is all over. There doesn't seem to be one out there.

The docs and nurses told me last time I had chemo they couldn't figure out why I was so dizzy and lightheaded. I decided to recheck the side effects of the drugs I'm taking.

At least two of the four had dizziness and lightheadness as side effects. I didn't check the other two. At least I don't feel so crazy now.

That's about it for now. Hope all is well there.

Love,

Nancy

Subj: Better
Date: 3/17/01

Dear Ruth,

My grandmother always loved the new lambs in the spring. She always had one or two that she hand fed. Have you had any twins yet?

I read your book yesterday. I found it very interesting. I'll send it back this week.

I'm feeling better. It was a rough week. I thought I had an infection in the Hickman catheter. I've had a fever for 6 days (low grade), but they put me on antibiotics and every day it seems to spike in the pm, but everyday is a little lower.

I'm trying to get organized from my extended "vacation." A friend of mine is going to schedule my friends to help with meals, shopping, laundry and transportation in May. I think I'll be well taken care of. I think I mostly need to get Hope and Cole to pitch in a little more.

Hope went to the beach with one of her friends this weekend (they were off Thursday and Friday). Cole has been having a great time having friends over and going to his friends' houses and, of course, the college B'ball tournaments are on too.

Guess I don't have much exciting to report. Hope all is well there.

Love,

Nancy

Subj: Update on Nancy
Date: 4/3/01

Dear Friends and Family,

This is the first in a series of correspondences I will be sending you to update you on Nancy's progress with the stem cell transplant program at Duke. There are two attached letters to this message. The first is a letter written by Susan Grosslight, Nancy's younger sister. The letter provides an excellent description of the details of Nancy's treatment plan and some of the things Nancy will be going through. The second letter describes a simple means of showing support for Nancy during her challenge ahead.

Nancy went to Duke yesterday for the "apheresis" procedure whereby her stem cells were removed from her blood as described in Susan's letter. The good news is that they were able to collect enough stem cells that she doesn't have to go back to Duke this week for more "harvesting". Given that Duke just won the NCAA basketball championship last night, we are greatly relieved that we don't have to weave through bonfires to get to the hospital. As of today, we are still on schedule for Nancy to check into Duke on April 8th.

In closing, we appreciate all the support we have received from friends and family such as yourself. Thank you.

Best regards,

Jason

Nancy's News

As you know, Nancy Caplan was diagnosed with breast cancer in December 1999. For a year she was treated conservatively, but the cancer did not respond. In January of this year, Nancy decided to undergo a Stem Cell Transplant at Duke Hospital in Durham. A Stem Cell Transplant is a type of bone marrow transplant. This is her hope to have a long-term remission from breast cancer and get back to her active lifestyle. Basically, Nancy's immature bone marrow cells, called stem cells, will be removed from her blood, she will receive very high doses of chemotherapy to kill the cancer cells and then the stem cells are given back to her. Now this sounds very simple, but actually, it takes many months to accomplish. This complicated process will be explained a little less simply.

Starting in January of this year, Nancy started receiving chemotherapy every three weeks. The purpose of this was to see if the cancer cells would respond to this type of treatment. She received chemotherapy every third Monday, spent most of the next two weeks on the sofa, in bed or at Duke. Then, the third week, she tried to catch up with Jason, Hope and Cole. Thanks to the help of her family and friends this winter has gone fairly smoothly!

In mid-March, Nancy had every test you can imagine performed to determine her suitability for the transplant and got the green light to go ahead. So, her real battle begins the last week of March. Since Nancy has healthy bone marrow, she will first have to take Neupogen, a medication given under the skin that will stimulate her bone marrow to make extra stem cells. She will take this medication for several days in high doses. The first week of April, Nancy will have to undergo apheresis. This is a process that takes her blood out of her body, separates the stem cells for the later use and returns the rest of her blood to her. It is sort of like hemodialysis, but instead of taking out the waste products, it takes out just the stem cells. These stem cells are frozen and stored for the next two weeks until it is time for the actual transplant. Nancy will go to Duke each day for the 8-hour procedure and then return home at night.

On April 8, Nancy will enter Duke hospital for the next phase of treatment as an inpatient. The most intense part of the treatment will last about a week. This phase involves five days of very intense chemotherapy to kill all the cancer cells. The problem is not only are the cancer cells killed, but also the bone marrow so the bone marrow must be restored. In this extremely vulnerable time Nancy will not have any functioning bone marrow. This means her body will not be able to replace any blood lost. She will also be suffering the usual side effects of aggressive chemotherapy. After a week in the hospital, Nancy anticipates being transferred to an apartment minutes away from Duke Hospital to begin her recovery.

If all goes according to plan, April 16 will be the big day! Nancy will receive her previously frozen stem cells intravenously. Over the next two to three weeks, the stem cells will find their way into Nancy's bone marrow and start to grow new blood cells. During this time she will visit the Bone Marrow Clinic at Duke daily for treatment, including transfusion of blood and blood products, antibiotics, etc. She will be highly susceptible to infections and must remain fairly isolated from the rest of the world. She will be recovering from the side effects of the chemotherapy. Fatigue will be a predominating feeling. Each day should show a little progress!

Once her bone marrow has started to function again, Nancy will be discharged to home to continue her recovery. She anticipates this being around the first of May. It will take several months for her bone marrow to function normally again. This means several things. She must be careful about contact with people who might have an infection of any sort. Visitors to the house must not have infections of any kind. Trips out in public will be very limited for much of the summer. Nancy's energy supply will be very low and she anticipates lots of naps and relaxation. Regular trips to Duke for follow-up will be scheduled using what little energy she has. She will just plain not have enough energy to get anything done! (You know how active Nancy likes to be!)

During Nancy's time at Duke, family members will be with her 24 hours a day to provide care and support. Other family members will be at Nancy and Jason's home to help keep the family routine on track. Once home, family and friends will continue to offer support with meals, transportation (for Nancy, Hope and Cole), laundry, shopping, etc.

Nancy would like to build a paper "chain of support" for encouragement while at Duke. Cards mailed to Nancy's home address will be delivered daily. She will not be able to have any flowers or live plants while at Duke or for a while afterwards. Nancy is not sure when she will be ready for visitors, but will get the word out when it is time.

Once Nancy enters Duke, to keep friends and family up to date, Jason will provide information by e-mail. Also, there will be a message on the answering machine at home that will be updated every few days.

Nancy would like to replace the blood she uses during the month of April. If you wish to donate blood, please make an appointment at the local Red Cross and mention Nancy's name. They will be happy to take care of you!

Your positive thoughts, prayers and support are truly appreciated!!

Nancy's Chain of Support

Nancy is facing a very difficult battle against her breast cancer in April. While undergoing the Stem Cell Transplant at Duke Hospital, Nancy will be unable to have many visitors and will be fairly isolated from the world. To give her much needed support and encouragement, we are asking family and friends to create a "Chain of Support". It is easy to contribute to Nancy's chain. Simply cut a strip of paper 1 1/2" x 8 1/2" (You can just cut the bottom off of a piece of computer paper). Write your name and any words of encouragement you have for Nancy on the strip of paper. Send the strip of paper to Nancy's home. When it arrives we will connect your link to the last link of the chain in Nancy's room at Duke. We hope to loop it all the way around her room before she leaves!!!

Thanks for helping us build a Chain of Support around Nancy!

Subj: Nancy Update - Day 1
Date: 4/9/01

Dear Friends and Family,

Nancy's mom (Myra) and I checked Nancy into Duke yesterday (Sunday) at 10:00 am. After some initial tests, they actually set us free for a few hours. That was a big mistake! It was such a beautiful day, we almost didn't make it back. We had a nice seafood lunch at the Fishmongers restaurant in Durham, checked out Nancy's apartment (for next week), and strolled around the Sarah Duke gardens. The flowers were spectacular! We then checked Myra into a hotel conveniently located next to the hospital.

We then went back to the hospital and got Nancy settled in. I can't tell you how brave Nancy is being about this whole thing. It was hard to leave her last night but we could tell she was getting tired.

Today is a big day. She starts one of her "big" chemo treatments plus a thousand tests.

The support rings have been pouring in. Thank you.

Best regards,

Jason

Subj: Nancy Update - Day 3
Date: 4/11/01

Dear Friends and Family,

Nancy had her second day of chemo yesterday and, all things considered, fared pretty well. She is a bit swollen from all the fluids they're pumping into her body. As a matter of fact, they almost had to cut her wedding ring off but Susan came to the rescue and was able to finagle the ring off last night.

The stats follow: She had two bouts of vomiting, a low grade fever (100.7), blood pressure of 120/51 and lowered white blood counts (2,500). Nancy is participating in a study to closely monitor the metabolic rate of the chemotherapy agents in her blood. Consequently, they are taking a lot of blood samples to measure the concentrations of chemo agents still remaining. The theory is that by closely monitoring these agents, they can more accurately determine the appropriate dosage of chemo agents and minimize some of the toxicological side effects associated with those drugs. She is only the third person to participate in this study so it may take awhile to see the full benefits of this program. However, the doctors assured us that Nancy will benefit from this study since they can make immediate changes to the treatment protocol based upon the results from the blood work. Let's hope so.

That's all for now. I'll try to update you later this week.

Best regards,

Jason

Subj: Nancy Update - Day 6
Date: 4/13/01

Dear Friends and Family,

Today (Friday) is Nancy's last day of chemo! And none too soon I might add. She has been experiencing a fair amount of nausea the past few days so she is ready to move on to the recovery part of the program. If all goes well, she is scheduled to move into the Durham apartment sometime tomorrow afternoon. She will be more-or-less in isolation for the next two weeks except when she goes to the clinic every day for tests. She will get her stem cell transplant on Sunday or Monday (Happy Easter Nancy).

We want to thank each of you for the cards and support rings that you've sent. After I read them to Nancy, Myra and Susan then add the rings to the chain. Through Thursday, the chain has 232 links! It almost covers the entire wall of her hospital room! It's fun to see the nurses' reactions when they walk in the room every day and see the growing chain.

Some of you have enlisted miscellaneous groups (i.e. church, aerobics classes, work, school, etc.) to participate in the support effort. Since I do not have their email addresses, I would like to ask the lieutenants of these groups to please convey our thanks to the individuals who prepared such touching messages of hope. I really think it makes a difference.

I would like to wish each of you a Happy Easter. Thanks again for your kind words of encouragement.

Best regards,

Jason

Subj: Nancy Update - Day 10
Date: 4/17/01
Dear Friends and Family,

I hope everyone had a nice Easter. We did.

Nancy moved into the "isolation" apartment in Durham this past Saturday. Her sister Susan will do the lion's share of Nancy's care this week. She did a good bit last week as well along with her mother Myra. My nickname for Susan is "Florence" (as in Nightingale). Her other sister, Julie, cared for our children in Charlottesville last week and part of this week in Raleigh. Nancy's parents, Myra and Bob, will relieve Susan this coming Sunday and stay as long as necessary until Nancy gets back on her feet. My sister, Lisa, is coming to Raleigh on Thursday to help with our kids through Sunday. I'm basically the Cabana boy that brings things to people when they need anything (no drinks with umbrellas though).

Nancy had her stem cell transplant yesterday. Everything went as planned. She had no apparent adverse reaction to the carrier, which is good. Her white blood cell (WBC) count is very low which was anticipated from the chemo treatment last week. However, she is very susceptible to infections since she essentially has no immune system at the present time. Therefore, we are asking people to refrain from visiting Nancy in Durham until she comes home to Raleigh.

The WBC counts and other blood factors (i.e., platelets, etc.) should increase over the next two weeks as her stem cells grow. When these blood factors reach a certain level, Nancy can come home (Yeah!). She will still be very weak during this recovery period (1 to 2 months) so we are going to have to rein her in from her normal activities. Those of you who know Nancy well understand that this is going to be quite a challenge.

The support chain has grown to over 300 rings! Susan taped the chain to Nancy's apartment and it wraps around a good bit of it. I'll try to send a digital picture of the chain in a future update. Thanks to all of you for your contributions to this effort. Thanks also for the cards (I'm also the mailman). I read them to Nancy each night when I see her. She smiles at the cards and the support ring.

This is going to sound like a broken record but thanks again for all of your support.

Best regards,

Jason

Subj: Nancy Update - Day 13
Date: 4/20/01

Dear Friends and Family,

Nancy's recovery is coming along slowly but surely. Her white blood counts and platelets are still very low but that is expected. We are now waiting for the stem-cells infused on Monday to take hold (grafting process) and begin producing new blood factors (i.e., white blood cells, red blood cells, platelets, etc.) If things progress as we hope, these factors should start increasing over the next few days.

Nancy and Susan look quite at home in their new digs. They usually call the Cabana Boy (me) at work in the morning to bring them something at night (i.e., sweaters, food, dish-washer, dinette set, big screen TV, etc.) I'm going to need a U-Haul to get everything home! But as long as they're happy that's okay with me.

The support chain has grown to about 400 rings! It encircles the entire living and dining rooms of the apartment! I'll try to send you a digital photo when it's complete. The rings continue to pour in from all over the country. I'm going to task Cole with getting an exact number of rings for a week-end project.

Well, I'm off to see her now.

Best regards,

Jason

Subj: Nancy Update - Day 16
Date: 4/24/01

Dear Friends and Family,

I don't have a whole lot of new medical information to report to you regarding Nancy. She continues to go to the clinic everyday to receive various blood factors and fluids. She seems to be eating a bit more each day which is a good sign. She has experienced some low grade fevers over the past couple of days which apparently is expected. We are anxiously waiting for her white blood cells and platelets to start rising from their current levels. I spoke with the nurse practitioner in the clinic yesterday and she said it normally takes about 7 to 10 days for these blood factors to start rising. It's been 8 days since her stem cell transplant so we are still in the "normal" period. When these factors start to rise, I will send another update.

We had a nice weekend. My sister Lisa came down from Washington, D.C. on Thursday, April 19th, to help with the kids (and me!). We went to the ballet on Saturday night and saw a magnificent production by the North Carolina Ballet, North Carolina Symphony, and the Raleigh Oratory Company. Nancy's brother, Will, drove down on Sunday for the day to be with Nancy. Also present were Susan, Nancy's parents (Bob and Myra), Cole and me. Lisa took Hope to her soccer game (they won!) so they couldn't make the visit. We spent a good bit of time outside so Nancy wouldn't be exposed to any human bugs. We kept our visit short so we would not wear Nancy out. She was still pretty worn out when everybody left.

There was a changing of the guard on Sunday. Susan passed the baton to her mother in her role as Nancy's primary caretaker. Susan did a fantastic job as I am sure her mother will as well. Nancy's dad is helping me this week with the kids and the garden. I'm trying to get him to build a garage but I don't think he's sold on the idea yet. I'm still working on it.

In addition to our families, there are a lot of "behind the scenes" people who have been a tremendous support. Special thanks to Carole Gallagher, Sandi Raymond, Teri Hunter plus the people who have brought us meals, transported our children, planted flowers, sent notes and made phone calls of support. THANK YOU!!!

Best regards,

Jason

Subj: Nancy Update - Day 19
Date: 4/26/01

Dear Friends and Family,

Yesterday was like "Mr. Toad's Wild Ride" at the Duke Clinic. As soon as I arrived at the clinic in the afternoon, Nancy began shaking uncontrollably for the better part of an hour. (In the prior weeks she would throw up when she saw me so I guess this is an improvement.) Her fever rose to 104.2 degrees and she broke out in a huge rash all over her body. Needless to say Nancy's mom (Myra) and I were very worried so we gathered the doctors and nurses together to see what was going on. Apparently, Nancy had an allergic reaction to the antibiotics they were giving her through an IV drip. They stopped that immediately and gave her some Demerol which slowed down the shakes and some Tylenol for the fever. Her fever dropped to 103 degrees when we left the clinic for the isolation apartment at 5:00 pm. Her fever dropped to 100 degrees by the time I left the apartment at 7:30 pm and her shakes were mostly gone.

And now for some good news. As you know, her white blood cell counts were almost non-existent (i.e., less than 100) for the better part of a week. Yesterday they rose to 300 and today they were 1600! This is very good news because it appears the stem cell graft is taking hold. HAPPY BIRTH-DAY NANCY!!! We won't know how the treatment program is working on the cancer cells for several months but this is a very important step in the recovery process. Nancy may actually come home next week sometime, however, it will probably take a month or more before she can get around much.

Meanwhile, Nancy's dad (Bob) has been pretty handy around the house planting flowers and driving the kids to their various activities. Cole counted 454 rings this past weekend on Nancy's support chain! And they keep trickling in. Thank you.

We plan on having a quiet birthday celebration at the apartment tonight with Nancy's parents and our children. You may remember that we had to remove Nancy's wedding ring due to the swelling in her fingers, so I had the ring re-sized to fit her (courtesy of Haywood Poole of Land's Jewelers - Thank you Haywood). I'm going to offer her the ring tonight and ask her if she'll still be my wife. Wish me luck.

Best regards,

Jason

Subj: Nancy Update - Day 22
Date 4/30/01

Dear Friends and Family,

NANCY'S HOME!!! After a rocky beginning last week, Nancy made a remarkable comeback in the latter part of the week. Her white blood cell counts went from 100 on Tuesday, 300 on Wednesday, 1,600 on Thursday, 3,600 on Friday and 7,800 on Saturday! Normal range is something like 3,500 to 9,200 so she is in the middle of this range. So Nancy came home at 4:00 pm on Sunday to a yellow ribbon welcome, a pot of geraniums, and a welcome home banner courtesy of Carole Gallager, the Maudes, and Cole, respectively.

Her other blood factors (i.e., platelets, hematocrits, etc.) went up as well, just not quite as much. It will take a bit more time for these factors to get to normal ranges but that is expected. She is pretty wiped out from the whole ordeal so we are asking friends to give her some time (at least a week) before calling and visiting. My role has now switched from Cabana Boy to Mother Hen (although I still do the Cabana Boy stuff when requested).

Nancy's Hickman catheter was removed so she has no more tubes in her body. As she says, "I am no longer a Borg. Yeah!". She will have to go to the Duke clinic every week now for blood tests but she will get to receive these like the rest of us, with needles instead of the catheter (ouch).

With Nancy home now, my updates to you will be less frequent. I have enjoyed writing to you and keeping you informed of her progress. It was even somewhat therapeutic, particularly with the dozens of positive notes of encouragement I received from many of you. Thank you for those.

Even with this terrible disease, I told Nancy last night that she has received a tremendous gift. Most people go their entire lives and never know the impact they have on other people. Over the past three weeks, she has received over 500 rings of support, numerous letters, gifts, flowers, emails, and positive thoughts and prayers. I may nickname her Georgette Baily from "It's a Wonderful Life."

One last thing. The ring fit and Nancy said "Yes" to my re-proposal. Her judgment must be impaired from the medications.

Best regards,

Jason

Subj: Nancy Update - Day 40
Date: 5/18/01

Dear Friends and Family,

It has been awhile since I last wrote to you about Nancy's progress. She is recovering slowly but surely from the stem cell procedure. She continues to experience fatigue and nausea but those are normal side-effects of the procedure. She goes to Duke every Friday for blood tests. Her platelet and hematocrit levels are normal but her white blood counts are still a bit low. This is not unusual as I will describe below.

Shortly after she was released (escaped!) from the hospital, they had given her a drug called Neupogen which encourages the growth of white blood cells. A week or two after the stem cell procedure, they stopped giving her the Neupogen because they wanted her body to produce white blood cells on its own. At first the white blood cell counts dropped but now they are slowly increasing, meaning her body is indeed producing these cells on their own. This is good.

Nancy's primary caretakers over the past couple of weeks have been Susan and Myra. They are doing an excellent job of keeping Nancy on the positive recovery path. She is taking short walks every day which usually wipes her out. Her progress is easier to measure in weeks rather than days because the recovery process is so slow. Using this outlook, Nancy definitely appears better now than when she came home from the isolation apartment.

I am taking Nancy to the ballet this weekend so this will be her first major entertainment event since she checked into the hospital. Nancy loves the ballet because it makes her smile.

I would like to personally thank all of our kind neighbors that have provided our family transportation and meals during the past few weeks. The meals are so good I'm going to have to purchase a Nordic Track to keep my Mr. Universe figure intact (that comparison will definitely make Nancy and those of you that know me laugh hysterically).

Best regards,

Jason

Subj: We are back from the beach

Date: 6/19/01

Dear Ruth,

I 'm so glad you are back. Everyone was beginning to worry about you. Of course between all our travels and e-mails mix-ups, it's no wonder. I hope you get lots of orders. Would that mean you could get the bathroom back?

Sounds like quite a trip to LA. What other schools is Rachel looking at? I hear there are some pretty good schools in North Carolina.

I have to tell you a story about my roommate from college. She is second generation Japanese. She grew up in Maryland. She went to LA to visit her family there and they went to the beach. She said she felt very out of place. She finally realized that most of the people there were Asian American! (It's interesting that she now lives in LA).

We had a great time at the beach. Just what I needed.

More later.

Love,

Nancy

Subj: Nancy Update - Day 70
Date: 6/20/01

Dear Friends and Family,

It's been awhile since I wrote you about Nancy so I thought I would fire up a brief note.

Our family just returned from a two week vacation at Cape Hattaras. We had a marvelous time. We had a small encounter with Tropical Storm Allison for a couple of days during our second week but it did not dampen our fun. Nancy trudged out to the beach almost everyday (under her umbrella, of course), took walks, shot photos, organized a campfire on the beach and read 7 books! (I don't think I read seven books all last year).

She has a nice tan and looks terrific. Her hair is just starting to grow back and has the texture of goose down. I told her that she should keep her hair short if it stays this soft but she's having nothing to do with that. She would like to be hatless and wigless by Christmas.

We won't really know the efficacy of the whole program for many months so we are now focusing on the recovery process. Her latest blood work showed normal levels for all parameters which is very good. Nancy still has some side-effects from the chemo and stem cell treatment program including fatigue, nausea, and tremors. These should wane in time. She still needs encouragement to eat so I try to prepare meals for her when I can. Other people have helped when I'm not around.

I would like to thank our wonderful neighbors and friends for sending dinners to our family during Nancy's recovery at home. That relieved a huge burden from us. Thank you again Carole Gallagher and Teri Hunter for arranging the meals and transportation, respectively.

Best wishes to everyone for a happy and safe summer.

Best regards,

Jason

Subj: I might make it yet.
Date: 7/6/01

Dear Ruth, Every time I write you and e-mail, either someone needs me or I get too tired or the e-mail doesn't work.

Anyway, thank you so much for the wonderful box of goodies! We love the cookbooks. What a lot of work to do each of those. Jason looked at them and said, "I could cook from this. It looks so simple." I can't wait to try them.

I liked your books, too. Cole wanted to know the answer to "Why Projects Fail" and he didn't quite buy your theory. I think he thought he could use it for his projects at school. I think we need to read a bit more of it. Of course, yesterday he also wanted to know how many miles a person walks in a lifetime, how many steps they take and who makes the most money in the neighborhood with $2 million houses near us. No wonder I'm tired.

Thank you for the mixes. They are so handy when I want something fast. I can't go in the pool, lake or hot tub, so your bath salts lit off a light bulb that I can take a bath. Jason really likes the massage oil.

Tell Valerie "Happy Anniversary" and the same to you!

I am doing better over all, though this week it seems that I'm more tired. I think I am trying to do more and I'm not quite ready.

I go for tests next week. What joy.

Love,

Nancy

Subj: Hi!
Date: 7/23/01

Dear Ruth,

We had a nice weekend at the lake for Jason's Mom's B'day, though Lisa (Jason's sister) is stressed to the max. Both her sons have jobs away from home this summer. They are moving to Indianapolis, because John got a job there. She can't find a house she likes. She's worried about leaving her mother in Maryland by herself. Lisa has never lived more than a few miles from her mom. So she is a bit of a mess.

I got back my bone scan and some of the spots disappeared and some of the larger ones are getting smaller. We are very excited! Of course nothing is ever easy. Now they are thinking about doing radiation to my right breast. On top of that I didn't feel well, couldn't eat and had chills at the lake, so I called the dr. on Wednesday. He said get up here asap. They did a pulmonary function test and didn't find much, but they are afraid I might be developing pneumonitis (an inflammation of the lungs. It's a long term side effect of some of the chemo.) He put me on a high dose of Prednisone. Can't tell you how pleased I am. It will take until the middle of September to finish it. They still can't seem to cure the yeast infection in my mouth. My tremors are worse secondary to the Prednisone, so writing, typing and any fine motor movements are quite difficult. I am in amazingly good spirits. I guess that's because when I get tired (which is all of the time) I just lie down and read. I finished The Hobbit this morning. I had never read it or the trilogy that follows. So much for my tale of woe.

I did run in TJ Maxx to buy a couple of new things. You need different clothes for all these appts. Hope approved of all but one thing, she is my fashion consultant. She has a good eye for color and style.

I am getting out more. Hope is driving more. Cole has been at my sister Susan's. He comes home today.

I am going to attempt to find my pantry. I haven't really looked in there since March. Cooking around here is pretty minimal. Then I'll probably head for the hammock!

Hope all is well there.

Love,

Nancy

Subj: I'm not sure.
Date: 7/31/01

Dear Ruth,

Thank you so much for the copy of War and Peace. I've never attempted that. Hope I have enough brain cells left to process it! I decided to read Tolkien's Lord of the Rings series. I'm on #1. I read The Hobbit last week. After that it's on to Tolstoy.

I went to Duke yesterday and had another mammogram. It took 3½ hours. After all that my doc was out of town and the radiologist couldn't decide what to do with me. They are thinking about radiation to the right breast, as a precautionary measure. I've had enough. I'm getting in a worse mood every time I have to go there.

Hope is practicing being a couch potato. At least she's reading. She's about through Harry Potter's 4 books for the fourth time. Cole is having a great time with all his friends.

We go to my family reunion Thursday. That is usually fun. I haven't been out of Raleigh since June.

School starts August 13. I'm not ready yet. The summer flew by and we never got hardly any hot weather. It has been raining for a week. Today the sun is finally out. Guess I'd better get a shower before the natives get restless (Cole had one of his wilder friends over to spend the night.)

Hope all is well there.

Love,

Nancy

Subj: Hot
Date: 8/10/01

Dear Ruth,

It finally got hot here. Hope pretty much has to stay inside because of the air quality. Cole and I have been going to the pool in the late afternoon. I can't get in the water because of my transplant, but I just take a shower when I get home!

Cole and I went to "Meet the Teacher" last night. He rotates between three teachers. Hope had two of them in fourth grade. They are fine. I think he will finally get some more advanced math.

Last weekend the reunion was fun. It was nice to get out of town for a weekend. The best thing was my sisters and my nephew took Hope to the pawn shop guitar shopping. She's been saving her $ all summer. She found a beautiful one. Now I just have to find her a teacher. We agreed to pay for the lessons if she bought the guitar (Her idea).

I go to see the radiation oncologist next Thursday. I'm pretty sure I'm already signed up.

My tremors seem to be worse, probably just seems that way. I think typing is just as hard as writing so I'll make this short.

Hope all is well there,

Love,

Nancy

Subj: Doc
Date: 8/16/01

Dear Ruth,

I went to see the radiation oncologist today. After 2 hours, they told me I had a complex case and a thick chart. I almost burst out laughing. What would they think of Hope's chart? I guess the radiation dept. isn't used to chronic patients. You can only zap someone so many times. Anyway, he said he wants to wait until I'm off the Prednisone and then do a PFT and then start the radiation. (He said 6-7 weeks - 5 days a week). He said patients who have had high dose chemo can develop pulmonary problems from the radiation to the breast. (Actually I guess that goes for everyone). I'm taking a month off, I've had enough. I'm finally getting some energy back.

Hope and Cole started school this week and so far, other than a little too much homework, they seem pleased. High school agrees with Hope, though I'm hearing a little too much about "hot guys." Cole loves being the oldest at his school. They grouped them according to ability this year and he is very pleased. Maybe he'll learn something other than multiplication tables in math!

Jason went fishing on his business trip to Vancouver and caught 20 salmon. I wonder how much business got done?

That's about it for now.

Love,

Nancy

Subj: Stuff
Date: 9/1/01

Dear Ruth,

We started out the week with Hope getting a terrible headache, which I knew was a migraine, but didn't want to admit it. I finally took her to the doc on Tuesday and they gave her some Imitrex, which is one of the drugs I use for mine. (Of course migraines are sort of like asthma, they don't like to diagnose them as such.) She says the meds make her head burn for 30 minutes, but then it goes away. Wonder what her body will think of next. I'm proud of her, she didn't miss any school.

Cole is playing as a guest player in a tournament this weekend on a soccer team that is the next level up (there are three levels). We always stick with the lowest level – recreational, because the other leagues are too intense. He had a game last night and only got to play for 5 minutes, but I think he enjoyed watching the game. We have another one this morning at 10. It's raining – Oh joy! This league plays in the rain – rec doesn't.

I found a guitar teacher for Hope! I'm so excited. I've been networking for 6 weeks to find one. Every time I thought I had found one, the person recommending them would say, "We love him, but he's moving out of town" . This one is just moving into town. It seems like Hope and Cole have a lot of after-school activities this year, but I decided they were getting old enough to handle it and they were missing some things they really wanted to learn.

I'm confused about Rachel's educational status. Did she pass her GED and is she now enrolled in college? Chemo brain strikes again.

I have a lot more energy. I picked out wallpaper for the bathrooms and the kitchen. I plan to strip at least one bathroom and let the paperhanger do the rest. He comes next week to give me an estimate. This is all left over from the replumbing last spring.

I found some flannel and I'm working on a flannel quilt for my Dad for Xmas. I thought he was going to take the one I made for Jason home with him the last time he was here. I also found beautiful chintz for recovering the sofa and making valances on the third floor. It was $2.50 a yard. It's pretty bold. It has a black background and huge multicolored flowers. Jason loved it. I had been looking all over Raleigh for flannel and the shops wanted $10.00 per yard. I said forget it. A friend of mine drove me to Charlotte to this great outlet. We found it for $3.59. Much better.

As you can guess from the length of this letter, the tremors are getting better. They are still there, but at least I can type better.

Hope all is well there.

Love,

Nancy

Subj: Busy week
Date: 9/5/01

Dear Nancy,

We have managed to confuse everyone about Rachel's schooling. She is a senior in high school. But by being home schooled, she will not get a diploma. UCLA, on the other hand, does not understand this, and says that she has to have a diploma. So logically she would need to take the GED. We suspected, and rightly so, that she could pass the GED way before she was done with her senior year, so we had her take it this summer. That way, we thought that we would comply with UCLA and show them that she got a diploma early. She has already gotten one graduation gift, so you are among friends in your confusion. So sorry. She says that she is pleased to have the diploma, it gives her some relief. Bob is now wondering why everyone doesn't just drop out in about 11th grade, take the GED and get on with life.

We are working on getting some radio interviews. We have been getting a little pamphlet together, and of course the last minute printing and production problems have been a bit overwhelming. We got it done, and now I have to go back through my in-basket and see what I forgot to do. Bob says that he would like to be supported by a rich wife! We will see if anything comes of it.

We plan to go to Columbus on Sunday to pick up a chair, and deliver Valerie's wedding dress. She said that she would like to have it, so I finally got around to taking it to the cleaners to be boxed up. I had stuck it into the back of a closet.

My parents are cruising past Iceland now. They seem to be enjoying themselves. The are continuing to communicate via e-mail, so it really doesn't seem like they are gone. My uncle is going to teach again this fall, part-time. He enjoys teaching quite a bit. This summer he started camping so that he could save money on his trips. He has a little tent, a really short cot, and his bicycle that all go into his mini-van.

It sounds like you are getting stronger all of the time.

Have you considered caffeine problems when thinking about Hope's headache? We find that if we miss our regular caffeine amount we get what amounts to a migraine. Probably you already thought about that though.

Much love,

Ruth

Subj: What a week
Date: 9/19/01

Dear Ruth,

Thank you so much for the box of goodies. The pear bath salts look intriguing and the liquid soap smells divine. The mixes come in handy. Jason and Cole are all over the honey and apple honey butter. Thanks for thinking of us.

Hope says she's coming to visit if you have Sanrio merchandise. She especially likes ChocoCat and the packages of little stickers. There are like a hundred per pack and some of them are scented. I like the angel bear and bought a lot of the toiletry things for Hope last year for Christmas – like the spray bottle, the mirror, toothbrush and pill box. I think there was even an eyebrow brush. Our very most favorite thing is the new dollhouses. We both decided we were a little too old.

I finally got a new refrigerator, after lots of shopping and debate on which one would fit in the space we have. It is a GE and it's wonderful. We had the one we had in Ohio – a Kenmore. It never worked right and Jason needed one at the lab for lunches and such, so he bought my old one. What a clean-up job that was! No one had attempted to clean the old one since last January.

I stripped the wallpaper in the kitchen and two bathrooms. This is still left over from the re-plumbing job. I got a guy in for an estimate. He wanted $1400 to paper the three rooms (which includes $500 for prep work and does not include the paper). I was very depressed. I thought I would have to do the wallpapering myself. I thought that price was highway robbery. Even though I love to wallpaper I just don't have the energy or the patience to do it yet. I had a woman here this week. She said if I prepped the walls, she'd do it for $400. That was more like it. I ordered the paper Monday. Hopefully it will come in soon and she can get started next week or the week after. Two of my friends are coming over Friday morning to help me prep the walls. They are all excited.

Today my cleaning lady comes. She does a great job. I told Jason I could probably do the cleaning, but it would take me a while. (The stock market is making us tighten our belts.) Jason said we should wait until I finish my radiation. I go tomorrow to get the scoop on my radiation.

I messed up my back either sewing or stripping wallpaper. I keep hoping it will get better quickly, before they decide to do a bunch of tests on it!

We tried a different medicine for Hope's headache and it worked. She doesn't drink caffeinated beverages. I keep telling Hope and Cole how hard it is to quit. She is having problems with her asthma this week, but she insists on going to school. She says her goal is to have perfect attendance this year. Not too realistic, but I told her it was a great goal.

Hope likes her guitar teacher. Cole is pretty happy being a fifth grader. He is very busy at school.

My friend, Carole, invited me to a brunch in my honor this morning with her bible study group. She said they have been praying for me for a year and a half and wanted to meet me. I wasn't invited to the bible study, just the brunch. They must think I'm a heathen.

We are all shocked and saddened by the terrorist attacks. We finally realized Cole thought terrorists and tourists were the same word. No wonder the whole thing had him so puzzled. All the pilots we know who work for American are safe. Jason flew to Victoria today. I'll be glad when he gets home on Sunday.

If you are running out of things to do we got lots of them.

Guess I'd better run. Hope all is well there.

Love,

Nancy

Subj: later
Date: 10/29/01

Dear Ruth,

The radiation is making me tired. Every time I sit down to e-mail to you something comes up or I get too tired. Everything is fine. I'll try to write tomorrow.

Love,

Nancy

Subj: Getting there
Date: 11/01/01

Dear Ruth,

I only have 8 more radiations tx's to go. They are really taking a toll on my energy level. I hear one recovers pretty quickly though after they are over. I leave for Duke at 6:40 am after Hope's bus comes and then I get home about 8:30. Thank goodness the radiation department is on time. I come home and take a nap and then try to accomplish something and then take another nap at 1:00. I am pretty useless after 7:00 pm.

I had several drs appts. They may or may not see a new spot on one of my ribs. Unfortunately the tumor marker is up over 1000, but now I'm being told they don't know what that means. Here's what I wrote to my brother.

"The doctor didn't map out a plan. He suggested I consider a Phase I study of a new antiagiogenesis drug. We talked to the nurse and read the consent form. They basically want to give me a drug no human, let alone any breast cancer patients, have ever taken, take several chunks of skin out of my arm and have me go to Duke almost every day. She said some of the mice in the animal study improved 'a little.' I THINK NOT! I'm not that desperate, yet.

I guess my choices are other hormones, another antiagiogenesis drug such as thalidomide (sp?) or chemo. I think I'd like to keep the chemo in reserve for if/when it gets to my organs. Anyway I have 12 more radiation tx's left. They are wiping me out. It's like I took a giant step backward to July or so. I have a great suntan under my right armpit – very strange. The doctor is going to look at a few tests that he hadn't gotten a hold of and then he'll see me again in 3 weeks when I'm due for my pamidronate and I'll be finished with radiation.

Cole came home with his report card Tuesday and had all A's. He was so pleased. He tried all last year and had a teacher that just didn't give A's. All his teachers seem to like him. That helps. They wrote he is a role model for the other students. I guess we are doing something right with him.

Hope got her report card and got all A's and one B in geometry. Math is just plain hard for her. She somehow thinks other kids just "get" A's. I've been telling her some do, but most have to study and work hard to get them. She seems to get the idea now. Her goal is to be in the top 10% of her class. That's what UNC – Chapel Hill pretty much requires.

Jason is burning the candle at both ends and getting a little grumpy around the edges. He's just trying to get in some work.

My sisters are coming in two weeks to "help" me do some things I can't seem to get done. We usually have a great time, but don't get much done.

Hope and I are discussing plans for her 16th birthday party. I think I've convinced her to have one on the afternoon after their last exam. They get off at noon. She might even invite BOYS!

My friends have been making two meals a week for us, which is a huge help, because otherwise it seems that all I do is cook. I started my Christmas shopping today and got Hope and Cole's big gifts. I ordered a number of the books Hope wanted from half.com. Do you use that? I usually have all my shopping done by Nov 1 and wrapping by turkey day. Not this year. I think the word "simplify" is in order. I decided not to have a Christmas party for our friends. I'd rather sit home and play games with Hope and Cole (We rediscovered Tripoly last weekend when Jason was away) or watch a movie. What a party pooper!

Cole is about to get off the bus, so I better run.

Hope all is well there.

Love,

Nancy

P.S. What does Rachel want to major in?

Subj: <no subject>
Date: 11/21/01

Dear Ruth,

I'm on the run.

Have a Happy Thanksgiving!

Love to all,

Nancy

Subj: Re: Thanksgiving is over
Date: 11/26/01

Dear Ruth,

We had a nice Thanksgiving despite the fact my father was in the hospital over night on Wednesday with an inner ear infection. He came home in time for turkey. I wasn't much help. The fatigue continues to plague me.

Hope is still sick. I'm taking her to the dr for the third time. She seems to have a resistant sinus infection. She is truly miserable after being on Prednisone for 5 days. I keep trying to keep my patience. It's a trial.

I'm in the process of changing oncologists. I've never liked the one I had. A woman who does only breast cancer was recommended to me. I'll try to get in to see her soon. Meantime I have an appt. with the doctor tomorrow. He wants me to start weekly chemo. I just can't do it right now. I'm too tired. We'll see.

Jason is at the beach fishing and has offered to come home, but I think once I get Hope straightened out, things will be better.

Sorry to hear you may close the store, but I'm sure all the details get to you after awhile.

When is the Grand Canyon person supposed to get back to you?

Hope all is well there,

Love,
Nancy

Subj: Re: The job is postponed
Date: 11/29/01

Dear Ruth,

Sorry to hear about the job. Maybe you'll find something even better in a more exotic place like the Great Smokey Mountains in NC?

More later.

Nancy

Subj: Package
Date: 12/14/01

Dear Ruth,

WOW! What a bag full of goodies arrived here the other day. There was something for everyone. Hope proclaimed the Hello Kitty things "way cool" and has been alphabetizing the magnetic letters on the refrigerator. The soups and other mixes are so good. I especially liked the chicken noodle soup. The bread and the cake (was that stollen?) (SP?) are delicious. I love the jojoba soap and gel. Cole likes the snowman and will enjoy the hot pepper jelly. He likes things hot. We might let Jason try some of the things if he behaves. He is off to Montreal – not sure why. My short term memory is still bad and I can't remember things unless I see it written down. They say it is a side effect of the chemo.

Hope is home sick with a migraine. Nothing is helping. Not even the big gun drugs they give me. Today is her last day before exams. She should be at school. She wants me to drop off a few assignments that are due today, later.

I went up to Duke to get my monthly bone strengthener this morning and they now have one that only takes 15 minutes to give by IV instead of 2 hours. That was nice. I was back home before 10:30.

Cole's orthopedist said Cole's knee is much better and now he just has to keep up his exercises and wear his brace during sports during the next month.

My goal is to not visit any doctors for the next two weeks. I think it's possible.

I guess I'd better get up to school.

Thanks again for the box of goodies. Hope all is well there.

Love,

Nancy

P.S. Why Oregon?

Subj: We are back!
Date: 12/18/01

Dear Nancy,

We got into Fostoria at 4:05 AM, just 10 minutes late, pretty good for Amtrak. We had a nice, but tiring visit to New York. The odd leaving and arriving hours make me feel strange; Bob is very content. Anyway, the stores were very pretty and we shopped a lot, but didn't buy much. There were many other people shopping. On Sunday at about 5:00 PM we were descending to the main floor of Macy's and it was so thick with people that the woman behind us observed that you couldn't even see the carpet. Rachel said that she has never seen so many people in one place before.

She has chosen Oregon, I think, because it is a school and state that are fairly close to the home life that she has here. She will major in writing there.

I have to get serious about getting Rachel a Christmas present. We thought that we might find something in New York. When she realized that we were willing to buy her a gift, we were just entering Tiffany's. We said," no.",

Hope that all is well there,

Much love,
Ruth

Subj: Can you help me with my shoulder?
Date: 1/22/02

Dear Nancy,

When I was about 30 years old I leaned on my right elbow while lying on the floor, for about 20 minutes. When I got up, my shoulder hurt quite a bit, in the front of the joint. When I went to the doctor he gave me Motrin, and if you recall, I spent the next 6 months drugged out on Motrin. You were in NC at the time. Anyway, I finally stopped the drugs and babied the shoulder and it got better. Over the years I have adapted to it so that it would not hurt. I carry my purse on the left shoulder. I have my computer mouse on the left side, etc. A year ago I wrote out Christmas cards with a pen, and the shoulder hurt again. When it gets bad, I cannot carry even a piece of paper in my right hand without pain in the shoulder. If I baby it, it gets better. Lately there are times when it seems fine, then I do something simple and it hurts badly again. Currently, I can only write with a Flair pen, and cannot push the grocery cart through the store. So do you have any ideas of what is injured, and what I can do to heal it?

So enough about my shoulder. We are all in the February blahs here. Bob says that he will need a new pair of cowboy books to get out of it, and perhaps a new sweatshirt. I am a little concerned that the February blahs are here and it is only January. Rachel took yesterday off from home-school. I asked her today to write an essay about her thoughts about Martin Luther King, Jr. but she doesn't seem to like the assignment!

Rachel and I went out Saturday to a sale and got new towels for the bathrooms. Ours were fraying, and I nearly inhaled the fibers on one the other day, so we decided it was a health and safety matter! We were able to match the towels that we already have, so we didn't need to get wash-cloths and hand towels. They have some nice new desert colors out now, but our bathroom is pretty much black and white.

Hope that things are going well there.

Much love,
Ruth

Subj: Re: Can you help me with my shoulder?
Date: 1/23/02

Dear Ruth,

I've been thinking about your shoulder. Wish I was there. Do you have any tingling in your arm OR hand? Do you know what specifically sets it off? Do you take anything for pain? Is there a specific spot in your shoulder that hurts? If you can get your hands on a good anatomy book or Internet site, you might be able to figure out which muscles are the culprits. It seems the latest idea is to strengthen the muscles around the area of the pain when you are not in pain. Of course you have to be careful not to cause more pain. If you can answer the questions I might be able to help more.

I'm on my way to the Toulouse Latrec(???sp) exhibit at the Art Museum, but wanted to get back to you.

More later.

Love,

Nancy

Subj: Re: Can you help me with my shoulder?
Date: 1/23/02

One more question. Do you use heat or ice when it flares up?

Subj: The shoulder questions answered
Date: 1/24/02

Dear Nancy,

There is no tingling in my arm or hand. Pushing the grocery cart, writing with a Bic pen, leaning on my elbow, using a mouse with my right arm all set it off, along with the passenger side seatbelt if it pushes on it. I don't take anything for the pain. I do put my hand over it when it hurts badly and that little bit of heat seems to help. I try to do some arm curls with the little weight set, but generally have to stop after four or five with that arm. I found an anatomy book, remember I used to be a nursing major, and found what looks to be the site where it hurts. It looks like the joining point of the Pectoralis minor, and Coracobrachialis. I am sending you a box tomorrow and will enclose a Xerox page for you.

I got a bunch of books from the Grand Canyon Association yesterday, so now I have some reading to do. I had asked them for some examples of what they publish so that I would know what I was trying to mimic when I finally get the book to edit. We were all pretty excited to see the box, it doesn't take much to make us happy!

Hope that things are fine there.

Much love,
Ruth

Subj: Shoulder
Date: 1/30/02

Dear Ruth,

I've been trying to think of some sage advice to give you about your shoulder. I'll keep thinking about it. In the mean time, I know how much we hate docs, but you might see a sports medicine doc. Is there one in Findlay? I know you had a bad experience with Motrin, but you might try Vioxx or Celebrex. They are the new anti-inflammatories (sp?) You could try one for a very limited time (a week or so) and see if it helps.

I think your shoulder is just plain mad and finds any excuse to let you know. I wouldn't do any exercises that include resistance if you have any pain.

If you go to see a doc, I'd be hesitant to have anything to do with Prednisone – oral or injected.

Not much help. I'll keep thinking. My brain is slow and full of useless information.

Love,

Nancy

Subj: another question
Date: 2/4/02

Ruth,

If you lie on your back on the floor and put your arms out to the side and then bend your elbows and move your arms back, do you have the same range of motion in both arms?

Also, thank you for the wonderful box of goodies. Just what I needed. Hope is being 16 in a big way and I think we'll keep her, but it's touch and go.

Jason's mom comes on Thursday.

My uncle's wife died yesterday. She was 86. He is 90. She got up to get breakfast and fell back down on her bed and was gone. What a way to go. I liked her. She was a good person. I find little comfort in "She had a full life."

It will be a busy week.

More later,

Nancy

Subj: <no subject>
Date: 2/18/02

Ruth,

I'm still here. We had a nice b'day for my Dad. I'm trying to get the week organized. Hope is sick again. I took her in for blood work last week.

More later,

Love

Nancy

Subj: Whew!
Date: 2/28/02
Dear Ruth,

Thanks for calling. I'm fine. Just worn out. Hope missed 6 days of school and was pretty miserable. They couldn't decide if she had a sinus infection and bronchitis or walking pneumonia. She was on 2 different antibiotics and is finally feeling better. She's very crabby and has lots of make-up work to do. She is also pretty bummed because all of her friends now have "boyfriends." She could take her driver's test tomorrow, but she seems to have no interest in driving. She's not pleased because we can't afford to buy her a car. Jason and I think she's a bit intimidated by all the traffic and construction in Raleigh right now. I think we will keep her. But some days I wonder.

My parents were here to celebrate Cole's "Bridging Ceremony". He went from being a cub scout to a boy scout. We also celebrated his birthday on Tues. he is gong to have to wait a couple weekends to have his friends party. Scheduling is tricky with all the kids playing sports (soccer started) and Jason going out of town. I won't have ten 11-year-olds over here unless Jason is here. Can't imagine why.

Jason is doing the work of about 4 people and is getting a little grumpy. Hopefully some of these contracts will come through soon.

I am just pooped between Hope's illness and Cole's stuff and having company. I think I'm going to go back to bed for the rest of the morning. Overall I am feeling better though.

Hope all is well there.
Love,
Nancy

Subj: Busy
Date: 3/16/02

Ruth,

I'm fine, but busy, so don't worry. My sisters are visiting one at a time. I've had a lot of tests at Duke and they are going to change my tx. I'll know more on Wednesday. Sounds like – some radiation for a couple of spots on my spine and an oral chemo drug that won't make me lose my hair.

Much more later.

Nancy

Subj: Re: So how are things?
Date: 4/16/02

HI,

Nancy asked me to email you and let you know she would like to write, but isn't feeling very good. The computer is on the third floor and it is hard for her to get up here and sit at the computer. She is having radiation and she is nauseated and in pain, so once things settle from that she will be back to the computer. She is certainly thinking of you!

Susan

4/25/02

Dear Haags,

Wow! these surprises keep on coming! The blue nightgown & the other blue thing—(we think it's too pretty to call it a night-shirt) are just fabulous. I love everything about them especially the color, the weight, the fabric the size & did I mention the color.

I have to restrain myself from slathering on the "velvet creme." It is so luxurious & feels great. I love the smell.

On to my tale to woes

Last Wednesday night I couldn't keep anything down. Nothing

was coming out except my mouth. By Thurs. a. m. I was a mess & Susan took me to Radiation. They took one look at me and said that they wanted to hospitalize me. So 5 liters of saline, 2 pints of blood, a gallon of ginger ale, an enema, a foley catheter a bunch of morphine, an MRI chest Xray a visit to the urologist & a few other schemes they cooked up, I came home Sunday. It's a battle, but I finally feel better. What a mess!

My final radiation is tomorrow. What a nice B'day present! I get a vacation for a week a so & then on with the chemo.

Subj: Fine
Date: 6/7/02

Ruth,

We haven't disappeared. Just busy. We go to the beach Sunday for a week. More later.

Nancy

Subj: Re: Pictures
Date: 7/11/02

Dear Ruth,

Thanks for the pictures. Unfortunately only the last one of the cottages came through. They look "quaint." Are they? How big are the lots? Do you have lake access close by? I'm trying to imagine the other buildings, but having a hard time. Tell me again – my short term memory is still all messed up. Where are you going to live? Do you have a space for Haag Press?

WOW! Thank you for the crystals!!! They are beautiful and I think my window treatment idea will work. I found some organza ribbon embroidered with beads (flowers and vines) which I plan to attach to 8" wide tulle and then drape the tulle around the curtain rods and hang the crystals on that. Sounds a bit strange, at least it will be different and I should have about a million rainbows every sunny day. Now I just have to get to it.

I did get shingles last weekend all over one side of my scalp. It was very painful. I don't recommend them. After 10 days I can finally touch my head without screaming. What next? I'm having a hard time getting anything done. Crawling into a corner for a couple of days sounds good.

Hope has started working for Jason. She has been doing Greasefeast orders, but we decided I'd been tortured doing the business checkbook long enough and we should train Hope to do it. Besides my (home) version crashed and everything from 4/1 has to be inputted again. Yuck.

It rained very hard last night (after this drought) and our kitchen skylights are now leaking. Another project!

Life goes on. I'm going to my Mom and Dad's next Weds. for a break. Hope and Cole and I plan to spend a week.

Hope all is well there. Thanks again for the crystals. They are marvelous.

Love,

Nancy

Subj: More about the move.
Date: 7/16/02

Dear Nancy,

We went up to Lakeside yesterday and looked over the cottages more carefully. We haven't been able to close on any other properties because I let the bank pick the title company, and they picked a ditsy one.

The Sandusky lots are a little larger than the size of our lot in Findlay. We plan to live in one of the houses and have the office in the other. There is a room in the office building/house for Haag Press, much better than the bathroom that it was in! The Sandusky property is two blocks from Lake Erie; we have not found a swimming beach nearby yet. When we walk the two blocks to the lake, we can see the roller coasters of Cedar Point.

The Lakeside cottages are for the weekends. I don't know if we will be able to get them winterized this year, but next year we will have a year-round weekend place. The Lakeside lot is pretty small, like about 50 feet by 125 feet. The Lakeside property is five blocks from Lake Erie and there is a small beach for swimming. The cottages will have to be totally redone, but for now are livable. We don't like much of the furniture that is coming with the cottages, so will haul it back here and put it in with the auction that we plan. I imagine that we have nearly enough furniture here for all of the places. I think we may need a new bed or two. We are so excited about it all.

While we were in Oregon, someone came and asked the store clerk if we were selling the farm. The For Sale sign still has not gone up. They decided to make a big sign, and it has taken a while. I have been working with the gossip network, and that has produced one person who looked the property all over, and one phone call to the Realtor. I got a preliminary fact sheet for it yesterday and have it in the store now.

Rachel is all scheduled for classes and is pretty happy with Oregon. The state is very nice, we can't say much for North Dakota, however.

I have a lot of accounting, to make up for my time off, and then to prepare values for the farm equipment and store stock. Rachel says that we should go out to lunch, that sounds good to me!

Hope that you had a nice week visiting your parents.

Much love,
Ruth

Subj: This and that
Date: 8/23/02

Dear Ruth,

Hope and Cole are settling into school. So far no major problems with teachers. Cole didn't get the elective he wanted, so he's taking French. So is Hope. Hope is also taking Spanish III. I don't understand it, but she seems to really enjoy languages. Anyway, I remember enough French from high school that we are having fun speaking to each other in French.

We decided to quit soccer (yeah) and Cole is going to play on a tennis team. His first practice is tonight. Hope says she is going to start a running program. I'll believe it when I see it.

Hope has not been very happy lately. A lot seems to be connected to the fact that she doesn't have her own car (Most of her friends do). I was wondering if you had any words of wisdom on 16 ½ year olds.

Has Rachel left yet? I got confused about dates. I remember when I first met you one of the things you said was that "in 16 years I don't want to look across the room and see a man I don't know, and have nothing in common with." I think you accomplished that.

I'm doing pretty well. I find the nausea and the fatigue my most limiting thing. The shingles are much better. Just 2 small spots left. I get my next round of tests on 9/11.

Did I tell you we had a major leak in one of our skylights from a storm and that we have to have the kitchen ceiling, wallpaper and floors redone? (We hadn't gotten the floor done from last Spring when we were going to do it.) Our homeowner's is covering most of it. We have to leave the house for a week and stay in a motel. What fun. I've been trying to pick out wallpaper. I'm getting so I hate that job. I want a blue and white kitchen. Painted white above the chair rail and blue and white stripes below and use my blue and white plates for accessories. Everyone thinks I'm crazy. Jason won't let me start any house projects because I get too tired. He's right of course. It just makes me so frustrated!

How is your moving going? It must be a challenge to find things. I can't find things in 1 house, let alone 4!

Hope all is well there.

Love

Nancy

Subj: My thoughts about 161/2 year olds
Date: 8/26/02

Dear Nancy,

We leave with Rachel for school on September 26. Her classes start on Sept. 30. Everyone here thinks that she should have left already, so I suggested that we just keep her indoors for the next month! OSU starts about the same time, but the University of Findlay and Owens have already started.

Our moving is going fine. We have many things moved to Lakeside. Of course Sandusky has to wait to receive things until it is mostly done being fixed. Now we have problems with things that we want to be at Lakeside, but have to stay in Findlay until we move to Sandusky. The kitchen seems to be the biggest problem. We are doing Sandusky in stainless steel professional kitchen type stuff, and black. We are doing Lakeside in our antiques and white. Findlay was done in antiques and white. I have the new stainless steel and black coffee maker in Findlay, but we don't want to get too much stuff, because we still want the Findlay kitchen to look good while we are selling it. We keep making lists and packing things up and it seems to be working.

I do not believe in giving 16-18 year-olds their own cars. They are just not experienced enough and too many of them die that way. I think that I mentioned to you that, with Valerie, I told her she could not even drive alone after she got her license, until she had had about 250 near-miss accidents, with me in the car. Things like starting to go at a four-way stop and then seeing that the other guy is going too, and stopping. Or seeing that someone is running a stop sign and then stopping in time to not get hit. Or stopping in enough time when the person in front suddenly puts on the brakes.

That system was somewhat successful, but Valerie still had two small accidents on her own after that.

In your case, however, there is the other problem: you can't afford a car for Hope. So in this situation, I suggest that you sit down with her and go over your actual finances. I am not suggesting a confrontation, but a sharing of information. This much is coming in each week, this much goes out for food, mortgage, insurance, cars, gasoline, college savings, etc. We have had to do that over the years when the company has been having a bad year. It is amazing, once they actually understand that there is no extra money, and in fact a decision is being made each week as to if we can afford sandwich meat or not, they are able to withhold spending. We notice that our girls voluntarily didn't buy clothes at these times, even though we had allocated them a budget. So a real understanding of the money situation might help.

My last suggestion is one of those that I won't mention again. I think that you want, above all else, for your children to have a normal childhood. But I think that trying to create normalcy, in spite of what you are going through, may actually be stealing a bit from them. I think that they need to know, if they don't already, the reality of your illness. I think that they need to be included more in helping with the running of the household and family, that up to this point you have been doing on your own. Time spent cleaning, cooking, painting, assisting in projects with you will not only teach them how to do those things, but will give them time to be with you. Helping another is one of the most rewarding things a person can do. If Hope is asked to shoulder some of the responsibilities around the house, she will have less time to think about herself and what things she would like to possess. It is how you teach your children to handle life's problems that will best equip them to handle life. No one's life is normal. Dealing with what comes by is a great teacher, and also helps to bond people together.

Much love,

Ruth

Subj: Re: My thoughts about 16 ½ year olds
Date: 8/26/02

Dear Ruth,

Thanks for the advice. I needed a new strategy.

Love,
Nancy

P. S. today is our 24th anniversary. Hard to believe.

Subj: Old
Date: 10/1/02

Dear Ruth,

I'd like to buy a copy of Old Married Friends' Advice. How do I do that?

Nancy

Subj: Re: The book
Date: 10/2/02

Ruth,

Thanks.

Does Rachel have an address? I finally got around to getting her a graduation present!

I'm looking for empty plastic crates to put stuff in from the kitchen. I have to take a lot of stuff out and put it in the family room so the guys can sand the floor. What a job.

More later.

Love,

Nancy

Oct 02

Dear Ruth,

Thank you for sending the book.

We are back in the house, though the floors aren't finished Tomorrow - they are good at their word. I am doing the kitchen in blue & white. I have some willow ware & other blue & white china/pottery etc The wallpaper is going to be that white ceiling paper - It has a texture but no print. Below the chair rail will be blue (surprise!) I found a blue paper that looks like fine basket weave. I also have a nice border with some green red gold & blue (the background is white) I plan to stencil tile under the cupboards as a backsplash - Have you ever done that? I can't seem to find any directions for it anywhere. Then I'm going to hang up the plates & get a couple shelves, We found a great rug for under the table to help with scratches from the table & to reduce the noise. - but they don't make the right size.

Hope all is well & you can read this

Love,

Nancy

Subj: Thank you!
Date: 12/14/02

Hi Ruth,

Thank you so much for the roses! They are wonderful. Your timing couldn't have been better. We are having our Christmas open house tonight and they are going to be our centerpiece in the family room. Even my burly stud-man husband commented on how pretty they were!

I'm trying to get ready for our party right now but I just had to thank you first. I'll write to you more later this week.

Love,

Nancy

Subj: Re: Merry Christmas!
Date: 1/1/03

Happy New Year!

Christmas was not your Norman Rockwell scene. Cole and I both had a stomach virus that kept us on the couch most of the day. One of our friends brought Jason and Hope dinner. We packed that night and headed to D.C. and VA. To see families. I am wiped out! I go to Duke for tests tomorrow and to the dr. on Friday. Hope we can start 2003 on a good note.

Thank you for the wonderful box of goodies. What a nice surprise. I especially like the pie dish and holder and the man and the goat.

I'm gong to put in some more laundry and then go back to the couch to read and sleep some more.

More Later,
Happy New Year.

Love,
Nancy

Subj: disappearance
Date: 3/29/03

Dear Ruth,

Sorry I haven't written or called. They (the docs) decided to radiate my jaw because it went numb. Also my hips because of pain. I'm finished with that now, but I can barely eat or talk and I'm pooped. Jason is in British Columbia and my parents are here to help us.

More later –
Promise. Hope all is well there.

Love,

Nancy

P.S. How's the moving/selling going?

Subj: Wow!
Date: 5/16/03

Dear Ruth,

I am so bad at e-mailing you. I'm doing fairly well except for the fatigue and that I still have numbness on one side of my mouth. My latest time consuming task has been fighting our medical insurance company. Long story. They want us to change from Duke and we don't want to.

Cole is now a skateboard maniac. Only 2 weeks of school left. He is quite happy about that. Sixth grade was tough.

Hope is busy juggling friends daily, it seems. She is also playing her guitar and writing songs. She has really improved. We have to get on the college stuff. Neither one of us is very motivated. We need to visit some schools. Fortunately she has decided to go in-state so we don't have really long distances to travel.

I'm working on chair pads for in the kitchen and a simple swag for the window. I want to cut down the noise in there.

We go to the beach for 2 weeks beginning the 9th.

How goes the remodeling business and is Rachel coming home for the summer?

I certainly hope I thanked you for the wonderful Victoria's Secret crème. It smells divine. If I didn't – thank you.

Hope all is well there.

Love,
Nancy

Subj: Re: Are you there?
Date: 7/30/03

Dear Ruth,

Everyday I say to myself I've got to write to you and then I don't get it done. Since the beach we've been to Indianapolis to see Jason's sister, to the lake for the weekend with friends, and it seems a lot of other places. I spent last night in the hospital getting 2 pints of blood. This new doc I have won't let me get blood in his office.

We are having a family reunion this weekend. I'm going to Charlottesville tomorrow.

More later.

Love,

Nancy

August 26, 2003

Jason

Happy

Anniversary!

I could write "I love you, I love you" a billion times and that wouldn't touch how much I love you

Amy

Nancy

Subj: Re: How was your summer?
Date: 10/9/03

Hi Ruth,

This is Jason writing to you as Nancy's secretary. Thank you for writing to Nancy. She is very weak now so I am handling most of her correspondences. She is on oxygen now almost all the time. I read your letter to her and she laughed at the stories about your potential buyers annoying your neighbors.

Thanks again for your note. Tell Bob and the girls we said, "hi."

Warmest regards,
Jason (aka, Nancy's social secretary)

Subj: Nancy
Date: 10/28/03

Dear Friends and Family,

As most of you know, Nancy passed away last Wednesday after a four year battle with breast cancer. She was the most courageous person I've ever met. She never gave up her fight, even until the very end.

One blessing was that Nancy had a chance to say goodbye to our children, her siblings, parents, and close friends over the last few days of her life. I held her hand as she left our world so she was not alone, which gives me some comfort.

I spent a lot of time over the past week (and years) reflecting on the reasons why something like this happens. So far, I'm coming up empty. But I can tell you some positive things that I have observed. First, I have never seen a tighter family unit than Nancy's parents and siblings. No matter what was needed, they would be there to help. This has confirmed my faith in family.

Carole Gallagher, Nancy's "seventh" and best friend (and adopted sister) has earned sainthood as far as I'm concerned. The things she did for Nancy and our family are too numerous to mention but are much appreciated. The network of Raleigh friends that helped us through this crisis is a very long list indeed. I want to thank each of you for your meals, yard work, special projects, rides, and comforting words. This has confirmed my faith in friends.

In addition to our family and friends, I have observed numerous acts of kindness from doctors, nurses and other "strangers" in our lives. This has confirmed my faith in humanity.

So while many questions remain why something like this happens to someone as good and kind as Nancy, there is no question about the value that each of you has brought to our lives. Thank you.

Love,
Jason

Bye Nancy,

Hope all is well there.

Love,

Ruth

I found the following books to be helpful in answering my questions about breast cancer.

Ruth Haag

Bathsheba's Breast by James S. Olson (The Johns Hopkins University Press) looks at breast cancer through history. It gives a good perspective on this not-well-understood disease.

What Your Doctor May Not Tell You About Breast Cancer by John R. Lee, David Zava and Virginia Hopkins (Warner Books) is written by a medical doctor and a biochemist. It is a helpful look at the processes going on in the body during a cancer attack.

Breast Cancer Husband by Marc Silver (Rodale) gives good insight for those who are partners and helpers to a person with breast cancer.